Trim and Tone,

28 Day of Chair Yoga

for Seniors

The Complete Illustrative Guide To 250 Short
Seated Workouts for Strength, Flexibility, and
Balance in Just 10 Minutes A Day.

Francis Nova

Copyright © 2024 Francis Nova

Legal Notice!

This book is intended to provide general information and guidance on the subject matter covered. The author, Francis Nova, is not engaged in providing legal, medical, or professional advice. The content of this book is for informational purposes only and should not be considered as a substitute for professional advice. Consult with appropriate professionals for advice regarding your specific situation.

The author and publisher disclaim any liability for actions taken or not taken based on the contents of this book. Readers are encouraged to seek professional advice for their individual circumstances.

Every effort has been made to ensure the accuracy of the information in this book. However, the author assumes no responsibility for errors or omissions. If discrepancies are identified, please contact the author for clarification.

Thank you for respecting the copyright and legal rights associated with this work.

Table of contents

Introduction

"If exercise could be packaged in a pill, it would be the single most widely prescribed and beneficial medicine in the nation." - Robert Butler,

As people spend more time at their computers or on long trips, there is a push to include more physical activity into our daily routines. Chair yoga offers numerous benefits for our bodies, including improved flexibility, relief from cramps and stiffness, and a happier mental state. While it may not be your preferred workout, it is an excellent choice.

Chair yoga incorporates the same practice of the body moving through flows of motion and increased flexibility as traditional yoga cycles. Almost any traditional yoga pose or movement can be replicated and modified to suit chair yoga. Chair yoga incorporates pranayamas (breathing techniques) that can reduce anxiety, introduce meditation, and improve spatial awareness, in addition to increasing range of motion.

Benefits of Chair Yoga

The advantages of an active lifestyle are widely recognized and documented. It is commonly stated that "exercise is the best medicine." Fortunately, chair yoga is an effective and accessible exercise for anyone.

When you start practicing chair yoga, you will notice a sense of ease and relaxation spread throughout your body. Over time, you will notice that the tension that had previously accumulated in your muscles and joints begins to release, and basic daily tasks become possible again.

Using your chair for seated or balancing poses allows you to reap the many benefits of yoga, including increased circulation, feelings of well-being, and reduced blood pressure, anxiety, inflammation, and chronic pain.

Regardless of your limitations, chair yoga can help you feel stronger while also providing numerous other benefits. This comprehensive guide will benefit you in a variety of ways, positively affecting both your physical and mental health. Including:

Time-Efficient Workouts: Each session is designed to fit into your busy schedule, taking only 10 minutes per day. Experience the effectiveness of targeted exercises that yield results without requiring a significant time commitment.

Improved pain management skills: Researchers have repeatedly demonstrated that one of the perks of exercise is reduced pain. That is because working out prompts the body to release natural painkillers like endorphins. Chair yoga also helps you manage your pain. Other ways to deal with pain and discomfort include gentle movement, deep breathing, and imagining the pain leaving the body. The exercises and routines are gentle, simple, and designed to accommodate a wide range of mobility.

Holistic Wellness: Beyond physical exercise, our program focuses on seniors' overall well-being. You will engage in practices that not only improve physical strength and flexibility, but also promote mental clarity, emotional balance, and overall vitality.

Targeted Relief: Each day is dedicated to a specific area of the body, ensuring that you receive targeted relief where it counts the most. Our guide covers a wide range of topics, including neck tension relief, core strengthening, and hip flexibility improvement.

Improved Flexibility: Perform a series of stretches and movements designed to increase flexibility. Over the course of 28 days, your muscles and joints will become more supple, contributing to improved overall mobility.

Gradual Progression: The 28-day program has been carefully designed to provide a gradual and progressive journey. Beginning with basic exercises, you will progress to more complex movements, ensuring that your body adapts and gains strength safely.

Accessible Practice: Chair yoga is inherently accessible, making it appropriate for people of all fitness levels and mobility. You can do these exercises at home, using a chair as a support, which removes barriers to consistent practice.

Enhanced Balance and Stability: The program includes exercises that specifically target balance and stability. As a result, you will strengthen key muscle groups that are essential for maintaining balance, lowering the risk of falling, and improving overall stability.

Increased Energy Levels: Regular chair yoga practice can help you feel more energized. The combination of gentle movements and focused breathing helps to improve circulation and invigorate your body, leaving you feeling energized all day.

Better Posture: The program includes several days dedicated to posture improvement. By practicing proper alignment and engaging core muscles, you can improve your posture, reduce strain on your spine, and promote overall spinal health.

Joint Health: The guide features gentle movements and stretches that promote joint health. Incorporating these exercises into your routine will help to improve the flexibility and functionality of your joints, resulting in a more comfortable and active lifestyle.

Empowerment: The carefully curated routines will provide you with physical empowerment as well as a sense of accomplishment and self-efficacy. As you work through the guide, you'll likely become more in tune with your body and confident in your physical abilities.

Stress Reduction: Chair yoga has been linked to lower levels of stress. The mindful breathing exercises and relaxation techniques included in this guide are intended to reduce stress, improve mental clarity, and cultivate a sense of calm in your daily life.

Begin this journey with the belief that each day will bring you closer to a more balanced and healthier lifestyle. The advantages go beyond the physical, providing a holistic approach to well-being that is both sustainable and enriching.

Dispelling Chair Yoga Misconceptions

Chair yoga is often underestimated, and there are some misconceptions about it that prevent people from fully reaping its benefits. Here are some common misconceptions about chair yoga that we will address and debunk so you can see what it really entails:

Not Just for Seniors: It's a frequent misperception that chair yoga is only appropriate for elderly people or people with restricted mobility. Chair yoga is actually a very adaptable exercise that can be done by people of all ages and fitness levels. It is an inclusive and accessible form of exercise because it can be tailored to meet different needs.

Lack of Intensity: People who assume chair yoga is a less effective form of exercise may think it lacks the intensity of traditional yoga. On the other hand, by emphasizing controlled movements, isometric exercises, and strength building through a full range of motion, chair yoga can provide a surprisingly challenging workout.

Restricted Benefits: Another myth is that chair yoga offers less advantages than mat-based yoga. As it turns out, chair yoga offers a host of psychological, mental, and physical advantages. It's a holistic practice that improves flexibility, strength, balance, and relaxation as well as general well-being.

Not a Valid Yoga Practice: There are those who doubt chair yoga's validity as a legitimate yoga practice. Chair yoga is a legitimate, well-known form of yoga that has developed to accommodate people with a variety of needs. Traditional yoga tenets like breath awareness and mindfulness are incorporated, and poses are modified to be done with a chair for support.

Less Work: It's a common misperception that chair yoga is easier to perform than traditional yoga. The chair offers support, but the key elements are the use of muscles, breathing awareness, and the mind-body connection. It's a methodical and contemplative exercise that provides a mild but efficient workout.

By Dispelling these misconceptions, We hope to remove these myths and welcome you to the enlightening realm of chair yoga. It is not merely an adaptation of conventional yoga; rather, it is an accepted and worthwhile practice in and of itself, providing a wealth of advantages to those who accept its gentle yet effective methodology.

How to Effectively Use This Book

To get the most out of "Comprehensive Chair Yoga Program for Seniors: A 28-Day Guide," follow these tips:

Read the introduction. Thoroughly: Begin by reading the introduction to better understand the guide's purpose and structure. Learn about the benefits of chair yoga and how it can improve your physical and mental health.

Identify Your Goals: Take a moment to consider your personal goals and expectations. Whether you want to improve flexibility, gain strength, or reduce stress, identifying your goals will allow you to tailor the program to your specific needs.

Follow the Daily Schedule: The guide is organized into a 28-day schedule, with each day focusing on a different part of the body. To achieve gradual progression and optimal results, adhere to the schedule on a consistent basis. Each day builds on the previous one, resulting in a comprehensive and balanced practice.

Pay Attention to Considerations: Before beginning each day's routine, review the considerations listed in the introduction. These insights ensure that you approach chair yoga mindfully, taking into account proper posture, breathing techniques, and any personal limitations.

Listen to Your Body: Chair yoga is adaptable, and you must listen to your body throughout the practice. If a movement is uncomfortable or painful, modify it to suit your comfort level. This program is intended to be gentle and supportive.

Use the Illustrated Guide: The book includes illustrations for each exercise, providing visual guidance. Refer to these illustrations to ensure proper form and alignment, thereby increasing the effectiveness of each movement.

Incorporate Mindfulness: Chair yoga is more than just a physical practice; it is a complete experience. Pay attention to your breath, stay present in each movement, and cultivate an inner calm. This will increase the overall benefits of the program.

Celebrate Progress: Keep track of your progress over the course of the 28 days. Celebrate gains in flexibility, strength, and overall health. Recognize the positive effects chair yoga has on your daily life.

Share Your Journey: Consider sharing your chair yoga experience with others. Sharing your journey, whether it's with a friend or by documenting your progress, can inspire and motivate you as well as others.

By approaching this guide with intention and commitment, you will realize chair yoga's full potential and transformative benefits. Make each day a step toward becoming a healthier, more balanced, and rejuvenated version of yourself.

Considerations Before Starting

Before beginning the 28-day chair yoga journey, consider the following factors to ensure a safe and enjoyable experience:

Health Consultation: If you have any existing health conditions, you should consult with your doctor before beginning this chair yoga program. They can advise you on any changes that may be necessary based on your specific health status.

Physical Limitations: Take note of any physical limitations or injuries you may have. The beauty of chair yoga is its adaptability, so feel free to adjust poses to your comfort level. If you are experiencing pain or discomfort, speak with a healthcare professional.

Comfortable Attire: Wear loose, comfortable clothing that allows for free movement. This will improve your overall experience and allow you to fully engage in chair yoga poses without restriction.

Secure Chair: Make sure the chair you use is stable and secure. Place it on a non-slip surface to avoid accidental slips and movements. The chair should remain stable during the exercises.

Breathing Awareness: Throughout the program, concentrate on your breath. Practice mindful breathing, synchronizing your breath to each movement. If you become short of breath or uncomfortable, pause and resume normal breathing.

Maintain proper posture during chair yoga exercises. Sit comfortably in the chair, back straight, shoulders relaxed. Proper posture increases the effectiveness of the poses while decreasing the risk of strain.

Gradual Progress: Although the program is designed for 28 days, it is critical that you progress at your own pace. If a particular day's routine proves difficult, do not hesitate to repeat it before moving on. Consistent progress is critical.

Chair yoga focuses on the mind-body connection as well as physical movement. Approach each session mindfully, focusing on the present moment and your body's sensations.

Create a Quiet Space: Set aside a quiet, clutter-free area for your chair yoga practice. This setting encourages concentration and allows you to completely immerse yourself in the experience.

Hydration: Stay hydrated before, during, and after chair yoga sessions. Proper hydration promotes overall health and improves the effectiveness of exercises.

Consistency and Patience: The benefits of chair yoga require consistent practice. Commit to the 28-day program while keeping in mind that everyone's progress will be different. Be patient with yourself, and enjoy the journey.

Enjoy the Process: Chair yoga is more than just a physical workout; it's also an opportunity for self-care and meditation. Enjoy the process, savoring every moment of movement, and recognize the positive effects it can have on your health.

By taking these factors into account, you lay the groundwork for a safe, enjoyable, and rewarding chair yoga experience. Remember, the key is to listen to your body, make necessary adjustments, and approach this journey with curiosity and self-care.

Getting Ready for Chair Yoga

Prepare for a fulfilling chair yoga experience by following these essential steps:

Choose a suitable chair:

Select a sturdy, armless chair with a flat seat. To ensure a secure foundation for your practice, position the chair on a non-slip surface.

Clear your space:

Make a dedicated space for chair yoga by removing any obstacles around your chair. This gives you plenty of room to move and reduces the risk of accidents.

Comfortable attire:

Wear loose, comfortable clothes that allow for free movement. This will improve your ability to do the exercises comfortably.

Remove footwear:

To improve stability and connection with the ground, practice chair yoga barefoot or in non-slip socks.

Mindful breathing:

Start with a few moments of mindful breathing. Sit comfortably in the chair, close your eyes, and take slow, deep breaths. Center yourself and make a positive intention for your practice.

Proper posture:

Sit at the front of the chair, your feet flat on the ground. Maintain an upright posture by aligning your ears with your shoulders and hips. This provides optimal support for your spine during the practice.

Props (if desired):

Consider having props nearby, such as a cushion or blanket, to help you stay comfortable during certain poses. Props can add support and make practice more enjoyable.

Warm-Up Moves:

Begin the practice with gentle warm-up movements. Rotate your shoulders, flex and point your toes, and slowly move your neck from side to side. This helps to condition your muscles and joints for the upcoming exercises.

Awareness of the Body:

Take a moment to scan your body for any signs of tension or discomfort. This awareness will help you adapt poses to your specific needs and ensure a safe practice.

Focus on the Breath:
Focus on your breath throughout the practice. Breathe naturally and rhythmically, allowing your breath to enhance the flow of movements and promote relaxation.

Positive mindset:

Begin chair yoga with a positive attitude. Seize the opportunity for self-care and mindful movement. Let go of expectations and enjoy the journey, knowing that each session helps you feel better.

Following these steps prepares you for a rewarding chair yoga practice. Whether you're a beginner or a seasoned practitioner, the key is to approach each session with openness, mindfulness, and a desire to nourish your body and mind.

Week 1: Foundations of Chair Yoga

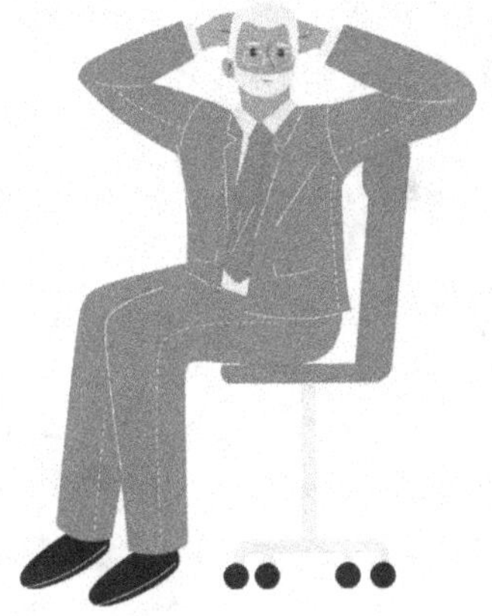

DAY 1: Neck, Shoulder, Arms, and Upper Back Relief

This exercise uses gentle movements and stretches to relieve tension in the neck, shoulders, arms, and upper back. Sitting comfortably in a chair, you'll perform controlled motions and stretches to promote flexibility and relaxation in these specific areas.

Guidelines for Performing the Exercise:

Begin by sitting with an upright posture.

Take each movement slowly and mindfully, coordinating it with your breath.

To avoid strain, practice gentle stretches rather than forceful movements.

If you feel any pain or discomfort, adjust the intensity of the stretches accordingly.

Perform the exercise on a regular basis to reap long-term benefits and improve upper-body health.

1- Seated Posture for Spinal Alignment:

- Sit comfortably in a sturdy chair, feet flat on the ground.

- Align your spine by sitting up straight and engaging your core.

- Place your hands on your thighs, palms facing downward.

2- Neck stretches:

Description: Gentle neck tilts, rotations, and stretches are performed.

Health Benefits: Reduces neck stiffness, increases flexibility, and relieves discomfort caused by prolonged sitting or poor posture.

- Slowly tilt your head to the right, bringing your ear near your shoulder.

- Hold for 15-20 seconds, feeling a gentle stretch along the left side of your neck.

- Repeat on the left side.

- Gently nod your head forward and backward at a leisurely pace.

3- Shoulder rotations:

Description: Includes shoulder rolls, lifts, and stretches.

Health benefits include reduced shoulder tension, increased range of motion, and improved circulation to the shoulder muscles.

- Lift your shoulders up to your ears and then roll them back in a circular motion.

- Repeat the movement for 15-20 seconds.

- Reverse the direction of the shoulder roll.

4- Chair-assisted arm stretches.

Contains wrist circles, arm stretches, and movements.

Health Benefits: Reduces tension in the arms, wrists, and forearms, promoting greater blood flow and flexibility.

- Extend your right arm straight ahead of you, shoulder height.

- Stretch your forearm by gently pulling back on your right fingers with your left hand.

- Repeat with your left arm.

5- Upper-back exercises:

Seated twists, upper back stretches, and spine elongation are all included.

Health Benefits: Releases tension in the upper back, increasing spinal flexibility and encouraging better posture.

Sit on the edge of your chair, with your back straight.

- Hold your hands in front of you and round your upper back, tucking your chin.
- Hold for 15-20 seconds, feeling the stretch between your shoulder blades.

- Return to the upright position.

Mindful breathing:

Inhale deeply through your nose, broadening your chest.

Exhale slowly through your mouth to relieve any tension.

Concentrate on the rhythm of your breath, paying attention to each inhalation and exhalation.

Guided meditation.

If you're comfortable, close your eyes and maintain a relaxed posture.

Inhale deeply and imagine positive energy filling your body.

Exhale to relieve any stress or tension.

Visualize a relaxing scene, such as a tranquil garden or a serene beach.

Remember to listen to your body, and if any movement causes discomfort, modify or skip the exercise.

DAY 2: Glutes, Lower Back, and Knees Strengthening

Guidelines for Performing the Exercise:

Sit comfortably with proper posture, keeping your feet flat on the floor.

Each movement should be performed with precision and purpose.

Throughout the exercise, make sure to engage the targeted muscles.

Gradually increase the intensity as your strength improves, but avoid overtraining.

If you have existing knee problems, do the exercises in a pain-free range of motion.

6- Seated Glute Squeeze:

Exercises include seated leg lifts, hip squeezes, and glute contractions.

Health Benefits: Tone and strengthen gluteal muscles, promoting hip stability and improving overall posture.

- Sit tall, feet flat on the floor.

- Squeeze your glutes together for 5 seconds.

- Repeat for ten repetitions.

- Gradually increase the duration of the squeeze as you become more comfortable.

7- Pelvic tilts for the lower back.

Description: Includes seated back extensions, pelvic tilts, and gentle twists.

Health Benefits: Targets the muscles in the lower back, increasing strength and improving spinal support.

- Sit comfortably with a straight back.

- Inhale as you arch your lower back and push your pelvis forward.

- Exhale as you round your lower back and tuck your pelvis.

- Repeat for ten controlled repetitions.

8- Knee lifts:

Exercises include seated knee lifts, leg extensions, and isometric knee contractions.

Health Benefits: Strengthens the muscles around the knees, improving joint stability and overall knee support.

- Sit upright and engage your core.

- Lift your right knee to your chest and hold for a moment.

- Lower it with control.

- Repeat with the left knee.

- Perform ten lifts on each leg.

9- Seated Marching:

- In a marching motion, lift your right knee first, then the left.

- Maintain a steady pace for one minute.

- Maintain a straight back and engage your core muscles.

10- Chair squats for glutes and knees.

- Stand in front of the chair, feet hip-width apart.

- Lower your body toward the chair as if sitting.

- Hover just above the seat and then stand back up.

- Perform 10-15 squats, keeping your knees aligned with your ankles.

11- Seated Cat-Cow Stretch for Lower Back

- Sit on the edge of the chair with your back straight.

- Inhale, arching your back and raising your chest.

- Exhale by rounding your back and tucking your chin.

- Repeat for ten controlled repetitions.

12- **Chair leg extensions:**

- Sit with your feet flat on the floor.

- Hold one leg straight in front for a brief period of time.

- Lower it with control and switch legs.

- Perform ten extensions on each leg.

Remember to maintain proper form, and if you feel any pain, modify your movements or consult a healthcare professional.

DAY 3: Feet, Ankles, Hamstrings, and Quadriceps Care

This exercise sequence is designed to provide care and attention to the feet, ankles, hamstrings, and quadriceps. Seated in a chair, you will perform a series of movements and stretches to promote flexibility, relieve tension, and improve overall well-being in these specific areas.

<u>Health Benefits:</u>

Foot and Ankle Care:

Includes ankle circles, toe flexion, and extension exercises.

Health Benefits: Increases ankle mobility, improves circulation to the feet, and reduces stiffness.

Hamstring Care:

Description: This exercise includes seated forward bends, leg extensions, and gentle hamstring stretches.
Health benefits include increased hamstring flexibility, reduced tightness, and improved posture.

Quadriceps Care:

Description: Includes seated knee extensions, isometric quad contractions, and moderate quad stretches.
Health Benefits: Quadriceps are strengthened and stretched, which promotes enhanced knee stability and function.
Guidelines for Performing the Exercise:

Start in a seated position with your spine straight and your feet flat on the floor.
Carry out each movement with controlled and purposeful gestures.
Focus on mild stretches and avoid any movements that create discomfort.

If you have any existing foot or ankle problems, do exercises in a pain-free range of motion.

This exercise sequence for Feet, Ankles, Hamstrings, and Quadriceps Care is a great complement to your chair yoga practice. It targets particular areas prone to stiffness and discomfort, offering a holistic approach to preserving flexibility and improving joint health in the lower limbs. Regular practice can help improve mobility and overall well-being in these crucial areas.

13- Ankle circles:

- Sit comfortably, feet flat on the floor.

- Lift your right foot and turn your ankle clockwise, then counterclockwise.

- Repeat with your left foot.

- Perform ten circles in each direction with each foot.

14- Toe taps:

- Sit with both feet flat on the ground.

- Lift your toes and then tap them down.

- Repeat for one minute, alternately lifting and tapping.

15- Seated forward bend for hamstrings.

- Sit with your legs extended straight.

- Inhale and stretch your spine.

- Exhale, hinge at your hips, and reach for your toes.

- Hold for 15-20 seconds, feeling the stretch in your hamstrings.

16- Quadriceps stretch.

- Sit up straight at the edge of the chair.

- Grab your right ankle and pull it to your buttocks.

- Hold for 15-20 seconds until you feel a stretch in the front of your thighs.

- Repeat with your left leg.

17- Foot flexes:

- Sit with your feet flat on the floor.

- Flex your right foot, pointing your toes to the ceiling.

- Hold for a few seconds, then point your toes away.

- Repeat with your left foot.

- Perform ten flexes on each foot.

18- Seated ankle stretch.

- Cross your right ankle over the left knee.

- Gently press down on your right knee to stretch your outside ankle.

- Hold for 15–20 seconds.

- Switch to your left ankle and repeat.

19- Activate hamstrings with leg lifts.

- Sit with your feet flat on the floor.

- Lift your right leg straight ahead, engaging your hamstring.

- Hold for a few seconds and then drop with control.

- Repeat with your left leg.

- Perform ten lifts on each leg.

Remember to perform these movements consciously, maintaining a comfortable and controlled state.

DAY 4: Shoulder and Arms Mobility

This exercise is intended to improve shoulder and arm mobility while increasing flexibility and range of motion. Seated comfortably in a chair, you will perform a series of controlled exercises and stretches that focus on the shoulders and arms.

Health Benefits:

Shoulder Mobility:

Contains shoulder rolls, easy stretches, and mobility exercises.

Health Benefits: Improves shoulder joint flexibility, relieves tension in the shoulder muscles, and increases total range of motion.

Arm Mobility:

Description: Includes arm circles, wrist stretches, and controlled arm movements.

Health Benefits: Increases flexibility in the arms, wrists, and elbows, leading to better functional mobility.

Guidelines for Performing the Exercise:

Sit with an erect posture, back straight and shoulders relaxed.

Each movement should be performed with intentional and controlled actions.

Pay attention to your breathing, inhaling and exhaling gently during the exercises.

Adjust the intensity of the stretches according to your comfort level.

Shoulder and Arms Mobility exercises can help relieve shoulder stiffness, increase arm flexibility, and maintain general upper body mobility. Regular practice can lead to better posture, less muscle tension, and a greater sense of comfort in the shoulders and arms.

20- Shoulder rolls:

- Sit tall, arms relaxed at your sides.

- Roll your shoulders back and down after lifting them towards your ears.

- Repeat for 15-20 seconds, keeping the action smooth and controlled.

- Reverse the direction for an additional 15-20 seconds.

21- Arm circles:

- Extend your arms to the sides, shoulder height.

- Make little circles with your arms and gradually increase their size.

- Continue for 1 minute, then reverse direction for an additional minute.

22- Triceps Stretch:

- Raise your right arm upward and bend the elbow.

- Use your left hand to gently push on your right elbow.

- Hold for 15-20 seconds, experiencing a stretch in your triceps.

- Repeat with your left arm.

23- Flexibility of the wrist:

- Extend your right arm in front, palm down.

- Use your left hand to gently press on the fingers, extending the wrist.

- Hold for 15–20 seconds.

- Switch to the left arm and repeat the stretch.

24- Shoulders stretch across the chest.

- Position your right arm over your chest.

- With your left hand, gently draw your right arm closer to your chest.

- Hold for 15-20 seconds, feeling a stretch in your shoulder.

- Repeat with your left arm.

25- Seated bicep curls.

- Hold a lightweight object in each hand (e.g., water bottle or light dumbbell).

- Bend your elbows and bring the objects to your shoulders.

- Extend your arms back down.

- Perform 15-20 reps with controlled motions.

26- Dynamic arm swings.

- Sit with your feet shoulder width apart.

- Swing both arms forward and backward in a controlled manner.

- Gradually increase speed for 1 minute.

- Take a quick break and then repeat for another minute.

- Remember to do these exercises within your comfortable range of motion, and if you feel any pain or discomfort, adjust the motions accordingly.

DAY 5: Hip Openers, Knees, Upper Back, and Pelvic Release

This exercise sequence focuses on expanding the hips, caring for the knees, relieving tension in the upper back, and increasing pelvic mobility. Sitting in a chair, you will perform a series of mindful movements and stretches that target these specific regions, increasing flexibility and well-being.

Health Benefits:

Hip Openers:

Contains seated hip circles, hip stretches, and mild rotations.

Health benefits include increased hip flexibility, reduced tightness, and improved overall hip joint mobility.

Knee Care:

Knee circles, lifts, and moderate stretches are all part of the routine.

Health Benefits: Promotes knee joint health, increases circulation, and lowers knee stiffness.

Upper Back Release:

Description: This exercise includes seated twists, upper back stretches, and spine elongation.

Health benefits include reduced upper back strain, increased spinal flexibility, and improved posture.

Pelvic release:

Includes seated pelvic tilts, rotations, and moderate stretches.

Health Benefits: Increases pelvic mobility, relieves tension in the pelvic region, and improves general lower back comfort.

Guidelines for Performing the Exercise:

Start in a comfortable seated position, keeping your spine straight.

Execute each movement with controlled and deliberate gestures that are in sync with your breath.

Focus on mild stretches and avoid any movements that create discomfort.

Adjust the intensity of the stretches according to your comfort level.

Incorporating Hip Openers, Knees, Upper Back, and Pelvic Release exercises into your chair yoga regimen gives you a complete way to improve flexibility and relieve stress in important areas. Regular practice can help to enhance mobility, reduce stiffness, and provide a better sense of comfort in the hips, knees, upper back, and pelvis.

27- Seated Hip Circles.

- Sit comfortably, feet flat on the floor.

- Move your hips in circular motions, clockwise and then counterclockwise.

- Perform for one minute, promoting mild hip movement.

28- Knee-to-chest stretch.

- Sit upright, with both feet on the ground.

- Lift your right knee to your chest and hold it with both hands.

- Hold for 15-20 seconds, feeling the stretch in your hips and lower back.

- Repeat with the left knee.

29- Seated Cat-Cow for Upper Back:

- Sit on the edge of your chair, with your back straight.

- Inhale, arching your upper back and raising your chest.

- Exhale by rounding your upper back and tucking your chin.

- Repeat for ten calm repetitions.

30- Pelvic Tilts for Pelvic Release.

- Sit comfortably with a straight back.

- Inhale as you arch your lower back and push your pelvis forward.

- Exhale as you round your lower back and tuck your pelvis.

- Repeat for 10 controlled repetitions, focusing on pelvic mobility.

31- Seated Butterfly Stretch.

- Sit tall, feet together, knees bent out to the sides.

- Hold your feet in your hands and gently press your knees to the floor.

- Hold for 15-20 seconds, feeling the stretch in your hips.

32- Leg extension with knee flexion.

- Sit with your feet flat on the floor.

- Extend your right leg straight in front, then bring your knee to your chest.

- Repeat for ten calm repetitions.

- Switch to the left leg.

33- Seated Forward Fold for Upper Back and Hip Release.

- Sit with your legs extended straight.

- Inhale and stretch your spine.

- Exhale, hinge at your hips, and reach for your toes.

- Hold for 15-20 seconds, feeling the stretch in your upper back and hips.

Perform these exercises gently and steadily, focusing on your breath and remaining comfortable throughout each action. If you have any problems or discomfort, adjust the workouts accordingly.

DAY 6: Shoulder, Arms, and Wrist Exercises

This exercise routine is designed to increase mobility and flexibility in the shoulders, arms, and wrist. Seated comfortably in a chair, you will perform a series of controlled motions and stretches to relieve tension and improve range of motion in these specific regions.

Health Benefits:

Shoulder exercises:

Description: Includes shoulder rolls, easy stretches, and mobility exercises.

Health Benefits: Increases shoulder joint flexibility, reduces tension, and improves general range of motion.

Arm Exercises:

Arm circles, controlled arm motions, and dynamic stretches are all included in the description.

Health Benefits: Increases flexibility in the arms and elbows, resulting in increased functionality.

Wrist Exercises:

Wrist circles, flexion and extension, and moderate stretches are all included in the description.

Health Benefits: Increases wrist strength and flexibility, reduces stiffness, and promotes overall wrist health.

Guidelines for Performing the Exercise:

Sit with an erect posture, back straight and shoulders relaxed.

Execute each movement with precision and deliberateness.

Pay attention to your breathing, inhaling and exhaling gently during the exercises.

Adjust the intensity of the stretches according to your comfort level.

Shoulder, arm, and wrist exercises can help relieve tension, increase flexibility, and preserve general upper body mobility. Regular practice can contribute to better posture, less muscle tightness, and a greater sensation of relaxation in the shoulder, arms and wrists.

34- Shoulder Blade Squeezes:

- Sit tall, arms relaxed at your sides.

- Squeeze your shoulder blades together and hold for 5 seconds.

- Release and repeat 15-20 times.

35- Seated shoulder press:

- Hold one lightweight thing in each hand.

- Extend your arms straight aloft and then lower them back down.

- Perform 15-20 repetitions with controlled motions.

36- Stretch wrist flexor and extensor muscles.

- Extend your right arm in front, palm down.

- Use your left hand to gently press down on the fingers to stretch the wrist flexors.

- Hold for 15–20 seconds.

- Repeat the process with the left arm and wrist extensors.

37- Seated tricep dips:

- Place your hands on the edge of the chair, fingers pointing forwards.

- Slide your hips off the chair and lower your body.

- Push back up to the starting position.

- Perform 15-20 dips, concentrating on working your triceps.

38- <u>Wrist circles:</u>

- Extend your arms in front, palms down.

- Circularly rotate your wrists, first clockwise, then counterclockwise.

- Perform for 1 minute to promote wrist mobility.

39- Rotational Bicep Curls.

- Hold one lightweight thing in each hand.

- During the lift, curl your biceps and rotate your palms to face up.

- Lower the weights and rotate your palms to face down.

- Perform 15-20 reps.

40- Seated Wrist Flexion and Extension:

- Extend your right arm in front with the palm facing up.

- Use your left hand to gently press down on the fingers, stretching the wrist flexors.

- Hold for 15-20 seconds.

- Switch to the left arm and repeat for the wrist extensors.

Remember to maintain proper form, and if any exercise causes discomfort or pain, adjust or skip that particular movement. Perform these exercises with a focus on controlled and intentional movements.

DAY 7: Lower Back, Hamstrings, and Neck Relaxation

This exercise routine aims to relax and relieve the lower back, hamstrings, and neck. Seated comfortably in a chair, you will perform a series of gentle exercises and stretches to relieve tension and produce a sense of calm in these specific regions.

Health Benefits:

Lower Back Relaxation:

Sitting back stretches, pelvic tilts, and gentle twists are part of the routine.

Health Benefits: Relaxes the lower back, relieves stress, and enhances lumbar comfort.

Hamstring Relaxation:

Description: Includes seated forward bends, hamstring stretches, and leg extensions.

Health benefits include reduced hamstring strain, increased flexibility, and enhanced circulation to the lower extremities.

Neck Relaxation:

Description: This routine includes moderate neck stretches, rotations, and calming motions.

Health Benefits: Reduces tension in the neck muscles, increases neck flexibility, and has a relaxing impact on the cervical spine.

Guidelines for Performing the Exercise:

Start in a comfortable seated position, keeping your spine straight.

Execute each movement with soft and controlled motions, keeping a sense of ease.

Pay attention to your breathing, inhaling and exhaling gently during the exercises.

Adjust the intensity of the stretches according to your comfort level.

Incorporating Lower Back, Hamstrings, and Neck Relaxation movements into your chair yoga program will help you decompress, release tension, and promote relaxation in certain regions of your body. Regular practice can help to enhance comfort, reduce stiffness, and boost general well-being in the lower back, hamstrings, and neck.

41- Seated forward bend for lower back and hamstrings.

- Sit with your legs extended straight.

- Inhale and stretch your spine.

- Exhale, hinge at your hips, and reach for your toes.

- Hold for 15-20 seconds, feeling the stretch in your lower back and hamstrings.

42- Seated Twist for Lower Back Release

- Sit tall and cross your right leg over your left.

- Place your left elbow on the outside of your right knee and slowly twist to the right.

- Hold for 15-20 seconds before switching sides for a moderate lower-back relief.

43- Seated hamstring stretch:

- Sit with legs outstretched.

- Reach towards your toes while maintaining your back straight.

- Hold for 15-20 seconds while feeling a stretch in your hamstrings.

44- Relax the lower back using pelvic tilts.

- Sit comfortably with a straight back.

- Inhale as you arch your lower back and push your pelvis forward.

- Exhale as you round your lower back and tuck your pelvis.

- Repeat for ten controlled repetitions to promote lower back relaxation.

45- Neck Rolls for Relaxation:

- Sit with your spine straight and shoulders relaxed.

- Slowly tilt your head to the right, then roll forward, left, and back to the starting position.

- Repeat in the opposite direction.

- Perform 5–8 neck rolls in each direction.

46- Seated Cat-Cow Stretch for Neck and Upper Back.

- Sit on the edge of your chair, with your back straight.

- Inhale, arching your upper back and raising your chest.

- Exhale by rounding your upper back and tucking your chin.

- Repeat for ten controlled repetitions to promote neck and upper back relaxation.

46- Gentle neck stretches.

- Sit tall and gradually tilt your head to the right, bringing your ear to your shoulder.

- Hold for 15-20 seconds, experiencing a mild stretch along the left side of your neck.

- Repeat on the left side.

Perform these exercises with soft and controlled motions to help your body relax and release stress. Adjust every activity to your comfort level, and if you get uncomfortable, adjust or skip the exercise.

Week 2: Balanced Body Journey

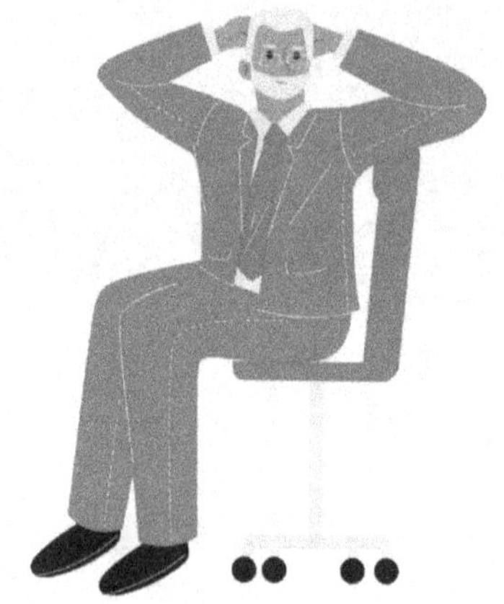

DAY 8: Hamstrings, Hip Openers, Quadriceps, and Upper Back Flow

This exercise routine aims to create a fluid flow that works the hamstrings, hip openers, quadriceps, and upper back. Seated comfortably in a chair, you will perform a series of coordinated motions and stretches to improve flexibility and relieve tension in these important areas.

Health Benefits:

Hamstring Flow:

Description: Includes seated forward bends, leg extensions, and dynamic hamstring stretches.

Health benefits include increased hamstring flexibility, decreased stiffness, and improved overall leg comfort.

Hip Openers Flow:

Description: This exercise includes seated hip circles, hip stretches, and mild rotations.

Health Benefits: Increases hip flexibility, relieves tension, and enhances mobility in hip joints.

Quadriceps Flow:

Exercises include seated knee extensions, isometric quad contractions, and flowing quad stretches.

Health Benefits: Quadriceps are strengthened and stretched, which contributes to enhanced knee stability and function.

Upper Back Flow:

Description: For spinal comfort, incorporate seated twists, upper back stretches, and fluid movements.

Health benefits include reduced upper back strain, increased spinal flexibility, and improved posture.

Guidelines for Performing the Exercise:

Begin in a comfortable seated position with an erect posture.

Execute each action in a fluid, rhythmic manner, in sync with your breath.

Concentrate on making smooth transitions between each piece of the flow.

Pay attention to your body's feedback and adapt the intensity to your comfort level.

Incorporating Hamstrings, Hip Openers, Quadriceps, and Upper Back Flow into your chair yoga program provides a comprehensive approach to increasing flexibility and releasing tension throughout the body. The harmonious flow improves general mobility, lowers stiffness, and creates a more fluid and comfortable movement experience.

47- Hamstrings: Seated Forward Bend.

- Sit comfortably in your chair, feet flat on the floor.

- Extend your legs straight ahead of you.

- Hinge at your hips and stretch forward to your toes.

- Hold for 20-30 seconds, experiencing a slight stretch in your hamstrings.

- Repeat 2-3 repetitions while inhaling deeply.

48- Hip openers: Seated Butterfly Stretch

- Sit on the edge of your chair, feet together.

- Allow your knees to fall outward, forming a diamond with your legs.

- Hold your feet and gently press your knees to the floor.

- Feel a stretch in your hips and inner thighs.

- Hold for 20-30 seconds and repeat as needed.

49- <u>Quadriceps: Seated Leg Lifts.</u>

- Sit up straight, feet flat on the floor.

- Lift one leg straight out in front, using the quadriceps.

- Hold for a few seconds before lowering it back down.

- Repeat with the opposite leg.

- Perform 10-12 repetitions on each leg while maintaining control.

50- <u>Upper Back Exercise: Seated Cat-Cow Stretch</u>

- Sit tall, with your hands on your knees.

- Inhale and arch your back, elevating your chest (Cow Pose).

- Exhale while rounding your spine and bringing your chin to your chest (cat pose).

- Flow between these two positions, synchronizing breath and movement.

- Continue for 1-2 minutes, aiming to increase upper back flexibility.

Remember to move slowly and softly while respecting your body's boundaries. If you feel pain or discomfort after a modest stretch, ease off and alter your actions accordingly. Prioritize your comfort and safety when doing chair yoga.

DAY 9: Lower Back, Neck, Shoulders, Arms, and Upper Back

This workout sequence is designed to promote harmony in the lower back, neck, shoulders, arms, and upper back. Seated comfortably in a chair, you will perform a series of conscious movements and stretches to increase flexibility, relieve stress, and promote balance in these critical areas.

Health Benefits:

Lower Back Harmony:

Sitting back stretches, pelvic tilts, and gentle twists are part of the routine.
Health Benefits: Relaxes the lower back, reduces tension, and improves general lumbar comfort.

Neck harmony:

Includes moderate neck stretches, rotations, and relaxing motions.
Health Benefits: Reduces neck muscular tension, increases flexibility, and promotes relaxation in the cervical spine.

Shoulder Harmony:

Description: Includes shoulder rolls, stretches, and mobility exercises.
Health Benefits: Increases shoulder joint flexibility, relieves stress in the shoulder

muscles, and promotes greater range of motion.

Arms Harmony:

Description: Performs controlled arm movements, dynamic stretches, and wrist workouts.

Health Benefits: Increases flexibility in the arms, wrists, and elbows, resulting in more functional mobility.

Upper-Back Harmony:

Description: For spinal comfort, perform seated twists, upper back stretches, and fluid movements.

Health benefits include reduced upper back strain, increased spinal flexibility, and improved posture.

51- Guidelines for Performing the Exercise:

- Start in a comfortable seated position with an erect posture.

- Execute each movement mindfully, paying attention to your body's responses.

- Coordinate the movements with your breathing for a rhythmic and relaxing experience.

- Customize the intensity to your comfort level, avoiding any motions that cause discomfort.

Integrating Lower Back, Neck, Shoulders, Arms, and Upper Back Harmony movements into your chair yoga program provides a holistic approach to general well-being. This sequence targets many areas of tension, producing relaxation, increased flexibility, and a harmonious balance in the lower back, neck, shoulders, arms, and upper back.

52- Seated Spinal Twist.

- Sit tall and turn your torso to one side.

- Hold the chair's back with one hand and the opposite knee with the other.

- Feel a slight twist through your spine.

- Hold for 15-20 seconds per side.

53- Neck Stretch:

- Sit or stand tall, lowering your right ear to your right shoulder.

- Hold for 15 seconds, experiencing a stretch on the left side of your neck.

- Repeat on the opposite side.

54- Shoulder rolls:

- Roll your shoulders back and down in a circular manner after lifting them towards your ears.

- Repeat for 30 seconds, then reverse direction.

55- Arm Strengthening:

- Hold onto the chair's armrests or sides.

- Lift your arms straight ahead of you, then lower them back down.

56- Upper back extension.

- Interlace your fingers and extend your arms in front, rounding your back.

- Lift your arms high and arch your upper back.

- Repeat this flow for 1-2 minutes to increase upper-back flexibility.

57- Full upper body stretch.

- Extend your arms overhead and clasp your hands.

- Lean gently to one side and feel a stretch along your side.

- Return to center and lean to the opposite side.

- Repeat for one minute to promote a full-body stretch.

Always move within your comfort zone, and adjust the intensity as necessary. This sequence is intended to strengthen your upper body while also taking into account the specific needs of your lower back and neck.

DAY 10: Abdominals, Hip Openers, Knees, Quadriceps, and Upper Back Revitalization.

This workout routine is intended to revitalize the abdominals, hip openers, knees, quadriceps, and upper back. Seated comfortably in a chair, you'll perform a series of energizing motions and stretches to improve flexibility, build strength, and refresh these important areas.

Health Benefits:

Abdominal Revitalization:

Description: This exercise includes seated core engagement, abdominal twists, and controlled abdominal movements.

Health Benefits: Activates and revitalizes abdominal muscles, promoting core strength and stability.

Hip Opener Revitalization:

Includes seated hip circles, dynamic hip stretches, and energizing hip motions.

Health Benefits: Improves hip mobility, decreases stiffness, and revitalizes the hip joints.

Knee Revitalization:

Description: Performs seated knee lifts, knee circles, and moderate knee stretches.

Health Benefits: Strengthens and revitalizes the muscles surrounding the knees, promoting joint health and stability.

Quadriceps Revitalisation:

Description: Includes seated knee extensions, flowing quad stretches, and isometric contractions.

Health Benefits: Activates and revitalizes the quadriceps, increasing strength and flexibility.

Upper Back Revitalization:

Description: For spinal comfort, perform seated twists, upper back stretches, and stimulating motions.

Health Benefits: Reduces upper back strain, increases spinal flexibility, and revitalizes upper back muscles.

Guidelines for Performing the Exercise:

Start in a comfortable seated position with a straight spine.

Execute each movement with deliberate and controlled gestures.

To get a harmonic experience, coordinate your breath with the exercises.

Customize the intensity to your comfort level, avoiding overexertion.

Incorporating Abdominals, Hip Openers, Knees, Quadriceps, and Upper Back Revitalization movements into your chair yoga regimen promotes general well-being. This sequence combines strength-building and flexibility-enhancing movements to refresh critical areas, producing a feeling of vitality and regeneration.

Focus on abdominals, hip openers, knees, quadriceps, and upper back revitalization.

This energizing sequence incorporates specific exercises for the abdominals, hip openers, knees, quads, and upper back to increase strength and flexibility. Follow these steps to complete a comprehensive chair yoga session:

58- Seated Knee Lifts:

- Sit tall and lift one knee to your chest.

- Hold for a few seconds while working your abdominal muscles.

- Lower the leg and repeat on the opposite side.

- Alternate 10-12 reps on each leg.

59- Hip Opener: Seated Figure-Four Stretch

- Cross one ankle over the other knee to form a figure-four formation.

- Gently press down on the crossed knee to feel a stretch in the hip.

- Hold for 15-20 seconds and then switch sides.

60- Engage quadriceps with seated leg extensions.

- Sit with your legs straight.

- Lift one leg, engage your quadriceps, and hold for a few seconds.

- Lower the leg and repeat on the opposite side.

- Perform 10–12 repetitions on each leg.

61- Seated bicycle crunches promote abdominal activation.

- Sit tall and bring one knee to your chest, While turning toward it.

- Repeat on the opposite side, resulting in a bicycle-like motion.

- Continue for 1-2 minutes while activating your abdominal muscles.

62- Upper Back Revitalization: Seated Cat-Cow Stretch

- Sit upright and alternate between arching your back (Cow) and rounding it (Cat).

- Flow through these poses to increase upper-back flexibility.

- Continue for 1–2 minutes.

63- Full Body Integration: Seated Mountain Pose.

- Sit tall, arms stretched aloft.

- Reach for the heavens, stretching your spine.

- Hold for 30 seconds to achieve a full-body stretch.

Always listen to your body and adjust the intensity to your comfort level. This sequence seeks to reinvigorate the core and entire body, providing a comprehensive chair yoga experience.

DAY 11: Flow for Upper Back, Hip, Pelvic, Shoulder, and Arm Harmony

This fluid workout pattern is designed to balance the upper back, hips, pelvis, shoulders, and arms. Sitting comfortably in a chair, you'll go through a series of conscious motions and stretches that promote flexibility, relieve tension, and build a sense of connection among these interconnected areas.

Health Benefits:

Upper-Back Harmony:

Seated twists, mild stretches, and flowing motions can help with spinal comfort.

Health benefits include reduced upper back strain, increased spinal flexibility, and improved posture.

Hip Harmony:

Include seated hip circles, hip stretches, and dynamic motions to improve mobility.

Health benefits include increased hip flexibility, reduced tightness, and improved overall hip joint comfort.

Pelvic Harmony:

Incorporate sitting pelvic tilts, rotations, and mild stretches to improve pelvic mobility.

Health Benefits: Improves pelvic flexibility, relieves strain, and adds to overall lower back comfort.

Shoulder Harmony:

Description: Perform shoulder rolls, stretches, and controlled arm movements.

Health Benefits: Increases shoulder joint flexibility, relieves stress in shoulder muscles, and promotes total range of motion.

Arm Harmony:

Description: Include flowing arm circles, controlled motions, and dynamic stretches.

Health Benefits: Increases flexibility in the arms, wrists, and elbows, resulting in more functional mobility.

Guidelines for Performing the Exercise Flow:

Start in a comfortable seated position with an erect posture.

Move smoothly through each aspect of the flow, synchronized with your breath.

Smooth transitions between upper-back, hip, pelvic, shoulder, and arm movements are essential.

Pay attention to your body's feedback and adapt the intensity to your comfort level.

Including the Upper Back, Hip, Pelvic, Shoulder, and Arm Harmony flow in your chair yoga program promotes general well-being. This continuous series develops bodily unity by increasing flexibility, relieving tension, and improving the interrelated harmony of the upper back, hips, pelvis, shoulders, and arms.

Focus: Harmony in the upper back, hips, pelvis, shoulders, and arms.

This flowing chair yoga sequence focuses on bringing harmony to the upper back, hips, pelvis, shoulders, and arms. Follow these measures to ensure a balanced and harmonious chair yoga session:

64- **Seated Cat-Cow Flow**:

- Sit upright and alternate between arching your back (Cow) and rounding it (Cat).

- Flow through these positions, synchronizing breath and movement.

- Continue for 1-2 minutes, aiming to increase upper back flexibility.

65- Hip and pelvic circles:

- Sit comfortably, then gradually rotate your hips in circular motions.

- Feel the movement in your hips and pelvis.

- Repeat for 1 minute and then switch ways.

66- Shoulder Rolls and Arm Extension:

- Roll your shoulders back and down after lifting them towards your ears.

- Extend your arms outward during the shoulder rolls.

- Repeat for around 1-2 minutes to improve shoulder and arm mobility.

67- Dynamic arm swings:

- Sit tall and softly wave your arms side to side.

- Engage your core and experience a slight stretch in your upper back.

- Continue for 1 minute with a smooth and rhythmic motion.

68- Integrated twists:

- Sit tall and shift your torso to one side, placing one hand on the opposing knee.

- Alternate sides to form a smooth twisting action.

- Repeat for two minutes to promote upper-body harmony.

69- Arm Flow: Reach and Pull

- Extend one arm overhead and stretch to the opposing side.

- Repeat on the other side, forming a continuous reach and pull motion.

- Continue for 1-2 minutes to improve coordination and flexibility.

Always move with awareness and adjust the movements to your comfort level. This sequence is intended to promote harmony and flexibility in the upper back, hips, pelvis, shoulders, and arms.

DAY 12: Psoas Muscle Release for Upper Back Comfort

This exercise is specifically designed to relieve stress in the psoas muscle, which improves upper back comfort. Seated comfortably in a chair, you'll perform focused motions and stretches to relieve psoas tightness and promote upper-back relaxation.

Health Benefits:

Psoas Muscle Release:

Description: Includes seated psoas stretches, mild tension-relieving motions, and mindful breathing.

Health Benefits: Reduces stress in the psoas muscle, which can enhance upper back comfort and spinal flexibility.

Guidelines for Performing the Exercise:

Begin in a comfortable seated position, keeping your back straight.

Perform gentle stretches that target the psoas muscle while paying attention to your body's response.

Controlled breathing might help to relax and relieve tension in the upper back.

Customize the intensity to your comfort level, avoiding any motions that cause discomfort.

Additional Tips:

Perform this exercise on a regular basis to progressively relieve tension in the psoas muscle.

Throughout the exercise, remember to relax and allow the psoas to extend and release.

Be aware of any sensations or pain and make adjustments as necessary.

Incorporating Psoas Muscle Release for Upper Back Comfort into your chair yoga program can help you achieve a more relaxed and pleasant upper back. By focusing on tension in the psoas muscle, you boost general spinal health and improve upper back comfort during your sitting practice.

Focus on Psoas Muscle Release for Comfort.

This session focuses on the Psoas muscle, which helps to relieve upper back discomfort. The Psoas muscle connects the spine to the legs and can cause upper back discomfort. To release your Psoas muscles mindfully, follow these steps:

70- <u>Seated Psoas Stretch.</u>

- Sit comfortably, feet flat on the floor.

- Slide one foot back and allow the knee to bend.

- Feel the stretch at the front of your hips and upper thighs.

- Hold for 20-30 seconds per side, breathing deeply.

71- Chair Psoas Activation:

- Sit up straight and work your core.

- Lift one leg towards your chest to activate the Psoas.

- Hold for a few seconds and then lower your leg.

- Repeat on the opposite side for 10-12 repetitions.

72- Seated Side Bend with Psoas Emphasis:

- Sit tall and extend one arm overhead.

- Bend gently to the side, accentuating the stretch in the Psoas.

- Hold for 15-20 seconds and then switch sides.

73- Mindful breathing for Psoas release.

- Sit comfortably, close your eyes, and concentrate on your breathing.

- Inhale deeply and allow your belly to stretch.

- Exhale slowly to relieve tension in the Psoas.

- Continue for 3-5 minutes to promote relaxation.

74- Seated Psoas Massage:

- Massage the area around the Psoas muscle lightly with your fingers.

- Use circular strokes with light pressure.

- Massage for 2-3 minutes, focusing on any areas of tightness.

75- Psoas Release Visualization:

- Close your eyes and envision the Psoas muscle releasing tension.

- Imagine warmth and calm radiating across your upper back.

- Spend 5 minutes with this visualization to allow for mental and bodily relief.

Always be cautious of your body's limits when performing these moves. If you feel any pain, ease off and adjust as needed. This Psoas release sequence aims to improve upper-back comfort and relaxation.

DAY 13: Whole-Body Wellness Chair Yoga Sequence

Wellness focuses on the abdomen, feet and ankles, hips, and lower back.

This session aims to enhance overall wellbeing by focusing on the abdominals, feet & ankles, hips, and lower back. Follow these instructions to have a complete chair yoga experience:

76- Seated Core Activation:

- Sit tall and use your core muscles.

- Lift one leg towards your chest and hold for a few seconds.

- Lower the leg and repeat on the opposite side.

- Alternate between 10-12 reps to promote abdominal wellbeing.

77- Ankle Circles and Toe Taps.

- Sit with your feet flat on the ground and elevate your heels.

- Circle your ankles clockwise, then counterclockwise.

- Tap your toes on the floor for one minute to improve ankle and foot wellbeing.

78- Seated Hip Circles.

- Sit comfortably, then gradually rotate your hips in circular motions.

- Feel for mobility in your hips and lower back.

- Repeat for two minutes to promote hip and lower back wellbeing.

79- Spinal Twist and Knee Hug:

- Twist your torso to one side and bring one knee to your chest.

- Hold for 15-20 seconds and feel the stretch in your lower back.

- Repeat on the opposite side.

80- Relax by practicing mindful breathing.

- Sit comfortably, close your eyes, and concentrate on your breathing.

- Inhale deeply, stretch your stomach, and exhale slowly.

- Continue for 3-5 minutes to promote relaxation and general wellness.

81- Seated Forward Bend with Reach:

- Sit with your legs outstretched, and reach forward to your toes.

- Feel a stretch in your hamstrings and lower back.

- Hold for 20-30 seconds to release tension in the lower back.

Always move mindfully, paying attention to your body's messages. During this chair yoga sequence, adjust the intensity to your comfort level and focus on your general well-being.

DAY 14: Core Activation and Relaxation Chair Yoga Sequence

Strengthen your abdominals, hips, knees, shoulders, and glutes.

This chair yoga sequence attempts to engage the core while encouraging relaxation. Follow these steps to have a balanced experience.

82- Seated Knee Lifts:

- Sit tall and lift one knee to your chest.

- Hold for a few seconds while working your abdominal muscles.

- Lower the leg and repeat on the opposite side.
- Alternate 10-12 reps on each leg.

- Seated Butterfly Stretch for Hip Openers.

- Sit on the edge of your chair, feet together.
- Let your knees fall outward, forming a diamond shape.

- Hold your feet and gently press your knees to the floor.

- Feel the stretch in your hips and inner thighs for 20 to 30 seconds.

83- Chair leg extensions:

- Sit up straight and stretch one leg directly in front of you.

- Hold for a few seconds to engage your quadriceps.

- Lower the leg and repeat on the opposite side.
- Perform 10–12 repetitions on each leg.

84- Shoulder Relaxation: Rolls.

- Roll your shoulders back and down after lifting them towards your ears.

- Repeat for 30 seconds, aiming to relax the shoulders.

- Reverse the direction for another 30 seconds.

85- Seated Twist for Core Activation.

- Sit tall and turn your torso to one side.

- Hold the chair's back with one hand and the opposite knee with the other.

- Twist and feel your core engage.

- Hold for 20 to 30 seconds on each side.

86- Relaxing neck stretches.

- Gently tilt your head to one side, feeling the stretch in your neck.

- Hold for 15 seconds, then switch to the opposite side.

- Repeat for a total of two minutes to promote neck and general relaxation.

Always move within your comfort zone, and adjust the intensity as necessary. This practice is intended to give a balanced chair yoga experience by alternating between core activation and relaxation.

Week 3: Harmony and Restoration

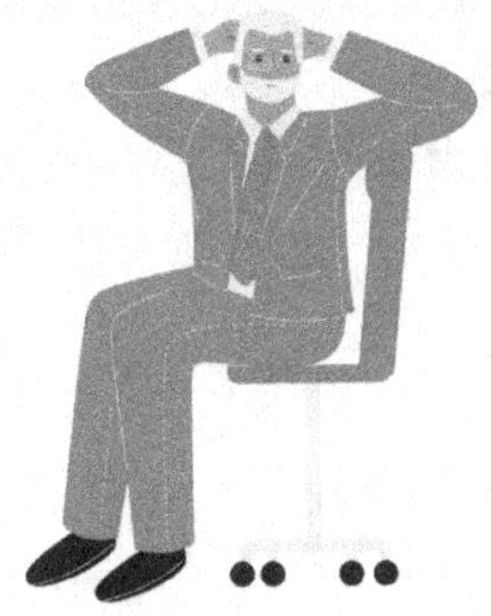

DAY 15: Hamstrings, Hips, Knees, and Quadriceps Care.

87-. Gentle hamstring stretches:

- Sit comfortably in your chair, feet flat on the floor.

- Extend one leg straight out, with the foot flexed.

- Hinge at your hips, reaching toward your toes.

- Hold for 15-30 seconds until you feel a slight stretch in the back of your thigh.

- Repeat with the opposite leg.

88. Hip-opening poses:

- Sit erect and cross one ankle over the opposing knee.

- Gently press down on the crossed knees to expand the hip.

- Hold for 15 to 30 seconds, feeling the stretch in the outer hip.

- Repeat on the opposite side.

89-. Knee Strengthening Exercises:

- Sit tall with one leg straight.

- Lift the extended leg a few inches off the ground.

- Hold for 10 seconds, activating the muscles surrounding the knee.

- Lower the leg and repeat on the opposite side.

- Perform ten reps on each leg.

90. Quadriceps Care with Mindful Movements:

- Sit in proper posture and activate your core.

- Lift one foot off the floor, bringing the heel to your buttocks.

- Hold your ankle in your palm and feel the stretch in the front of your thigh.

- Hold for 15-30 seconds, then switch to the other leg.

Tips:

Breathe deeply and consistently throughout each stretch and activity.

To reap the most advantages, perform the exercises slowly and steadily.

Listen to your body and prevent any painful movements.

Benefits:

Increased hamstring and hip flexibility.

Strengthening important muscle groups surrounding the knee to improve stability.

Quadriceps activation provides general lower-body support.

Improves blood flow and energy circulation in the lower body.

Remember to execute these exercises at your own pace, and if you have any pre-existing health concerns, contact a healthcare expert before beginning a new exercise program.

DAY 16: Feet and Ankles Renewal - Completing a Balanced Journey

Goal: Revitalize and care for your feet and ankles in order to complete a holistic chair yoga practice.

Session highlights:

91- Toe Tapping for Circulation:

- Sit comfortably, with both feet flat on the floor.

- Lift one foot at a time and tap your toes against the floor for 30 seconds.

- Improves blood circulation in the feet and ankles.

92- Ankle circles:

- Lift one foot off the ground and spin the ankle clockwise for 15 seconds.

- Then, rotate counterclockwise for an additional 15 seconds.

- Repeat with the other foot.

- Increases ankle flexibility and mobility.

93- Heel-toe Stretch:

- Extend one leg and flex your foot, drawing your toes closer to you.

- Hold your toes lightly for 20 seconds, feeling the stretch in the calf and under the foot.

- Repeat with the opposite leg.

- Stretches and relaxes the muscles in your feet and calves.

94- Arch Activation:

- Sit with both feet flat on the ground.

- Lift your feet ' arches to engage the muscles on the undersides.

- Hold for 10 seconds then release.

- Strengthens the arches and increases foot stability.

95- Full-foot massage:

- Use a tennis or small massage ball.

- Roll the ball under your foot, using mild pressure.

- Spend 1–2 minutes on each foot.

- Reduces tension and delivers a relaxing massage.

Tips:

Perform each movement slowly and deliberately.

To relax more, concentrate on your breathing.

If you are uncomfortable or in pain, reduce the intensity or omit the activity.

Benefits:

Improved circulation in the feet and ankles.

Improved ankle flexibility and mobility.

Relief from stress and soreness in the feet.

Completes the overall chair yoga experience by focusing on the foundation of your body.

DAY 17: Holistic Balance - A Full Body Journey

The goal is to achieve general balance and harmony throughout the body through a sequence of conscious movements.

Session highlights:

96- Mindful Body Scan:

- Sit comfortably in an upright position.

- Close your eyes and pay attention to every aspect of your body, from head to toe.

- Focus for a few minutes on your breathing and body sensations.

97- Seated Tree Pose Variation:

- Begin by sitting with both feet flat on the floor.

- Lift one foot and place the sole against the inner thigh or calf of the opposite leg.

- Place your palms together in front of your chest.

- Hold for 20 seconds while keeping balance.

- Repeat on the opposite side.

- Improves focus and balance.

98- Gentle Side Bends:

- Sit up straight and breathe deeply.

- As you exhale, gently bend to one side and reach your hand to the floor.

- Hold for 15 seconds then return to the center.

- Repeat on the opposite side.

- Stretches the side body and improves lateral balance.

99- Seated Twist with Core Engagement:

- Sit with a straight back and twist your torso to one side.

- Place one hand on the opposite knee, and the other behind you.

- Hold the twist for 20 seconds. Engage your core.

- Repeat on the opposite side.

- Enhances spinal flexibility and core stability.

100- Chair Mountain Pose:

- Sit with your feet flat on the floor and arms at your sides.

- Inhale and raise your arms upwards, palms facing each other.

- Hold for 15 seconds, then lift through the chest.

- Exhale and drop your arms.

- Improves general body awareness and balance.

Tips:

Concentrate on smooth, controlled motions.

During each pose, center yourself by breathing.

Modify positions as needed to fit your comfort level.

Benefits:

Promotes mindfulness and bodily awareness.

Enhances stability and balance.

Develops a sensation of calm and focus.

Combines the benefits of specific positions into a full-body experience.

DAY 18: Enhanced Strength and Flexibility

A well-rounded chair yoga session should include both strength-building exercises and flexibility-focused stretches.

Session highlights:

101- Seated Forward Bend With Resistance:

- Sit with legs outstretched.

- Wrap a resistance band around your feet and pull gently to your toes.

- Hold for 20 seconds and feel the stretch in your hamstrings.

- Improves hamstring flexibility and strength.

102- Seated Twist With Resistance:

- Sit tall and place the resistance band behind your back.

- Twist the ends towards one side while holding them in both hands.

- Hold for 15 seconds per side.

- Increases spinal mobility and engages core muscles.

103- Seated leg lifts:

- Sit on the edge of the chair with your back straight.

- Lift one leg at a time and stretch it directly in front of you.

- Hold for 10 seconds then swap legs.

- Quadriceps strength is increased, as is core muscle engagement.

104- Chair triceps dips:

- Sit on the edge of the chair, with your hands on either side.

- Slide off the chair by bending your elbows and lowering your body.

- Push back up to the starting position.

- Targets the triceps and increases arm strength.

105- Dynamic Seated Cat-Cow Stretch.

- Sit with your hands on your knees, arch your back (cow), and round your spine (cat).

- Repeat for one minute, moving between the two positions.

- Increases spinal flexibility and stretches the back.

Tips:

To avoid strain, perform controlled motions.

Breathe deeply and consistently throughout each exercise.

Increase resistance or repetitions gradually until you reach your desired level of comfort.

<u>Benefits:</u>

Increased hamstring and spine flexibility.

Increased strength in the arms, legs, and core.

Increased shoulder and hip range of motion.

Full-body engagement promotes general strength and flexibility.

DAY 19: Full-Body Empowerment

Objective: Empower your entire body with a chair yoga sequence that targets numerous muscle groups.

Session highlights:

<u>106- Dynamic arm and leg lifts:</u>

- Sit in an erect position.

- Lift one arm and the opposing leg at the same time.

- Repeat for one minute, alternating sides.

- Engages core muscles and enhances coordination.

107- Seated high knees:

- Sit with your back erect and raise your knees to your chest.

- Hold onto the chair's sides for balance.

- Do high knees for 1 minute.

- Strengthens hip flexors and improves cardiovascular health.

108- Chair squats:

- Stand in front of the chair, with your feet shoulder width apart.

- Lower yourself into a seated position without completely sitting.

- Stand back up, engaging your glutes.

- It focuses on the quadriceps, hamstrings, and glutes.

109- Seated Chest Opener:

- Sit comfortably and interlace your fingers behind your back.

- Lift your arms gently to open your chest.

- Hold for 20 seconds and feel the stretch across your chest.

- Improves posture by opening the chest and shoulders.

110- Full-body Stretch:

- Sit tall and raise both arms aloft.

- Extend your legs in front and point your toes.

- Hold for 30 seconds, stretching your entire body.

- Increases flexibility and relieves strain.

Tips:

Concentrate on smooth, controlled motions.

Throughout the session, pay close attention to your breathing.

Adjust the intensity according to your comfort level.

Benefits:

Full-body participation promotes general empowerment.

Increased heart rate and circulation.

Strengthening in the core, legs, and arms.

Improved flexibility and posture.

DAY 20: Fluid Harmony

The goal is to explore a continuous chair yoga flow that promotes fluid movement and body harmony.

Session highlights:

111- Chair Cat-Cow Flow:

- Sit with hands on knees.

- Inhale by arching your back (cow), and exhale by rounding your spine (cat).

- Flow through these exercises for one minute.

- Improves spinal flexibility and relieves strain.

112- Seated Side Bends:

- Sit with feet flat and arms stretched overhead.

- Inhale and lean to one side, feeling the stretch in your torso.

- Exhale and switch sides to create a smooth side-to-side flow.

- Enhances lateral flexibility and extends the waist.

113 Dynamic Seated Twist Flow.

- Sit tall and turn your torso to one side.

- Inhale back to the center and exhale, turning to the opposite side.

- Flow between these twists for one minute.

- Increases spine mobility while also engaging core muscles.

114- Seated Flowing Warrior:

- Sit on the edge of the chair, extend one leg back, and raise the opposite arm.

- Flow between sides to achieve a fluid warrior-like movement.

- Engages the core, strengthens the legs, and increases balance.

115- Chair Sun Salutation:

- Begin in prayer position, then extend your arms high before folding forward.

- Transition through a series of moves before returning to the starting position.

- Perform for three rounds.

- Promotes flexibility and energizes the physique.

Tips:

Maintain a steady and rhythmic breathing throughout.

Flow fluidly between movements.

Accept the flow of the exercise with grace.

Benefits:

Improves entire body coordination.

Promotes fluidity and ease of movement.

Increases spinal flexibility and key muscle groups.

Energizes both the body and the mind.

Objective: Take part in a relaxing chair yoga session centered on awareness and relaxation.

Session highlights:

116- Deep Breathing Exercise:

- Sit comfortably and close your eyes.

- Inhale deeply through your nose for a count of 4.

- Exhale slowly through pursed lips for a count of six.

- Repeat for 3 minutes, focusing on your breathing.

117- Seated Body Scan Meditation:

- Bring attention to each area of your body, beginning with your toes.

- Notice any tightness or sensations and let them subside as you breathe.

- Move slowly up your body, until you reach the crown of your head.

- Takes about 5 minutes.

118- Chair Pawanmuktasana (Wind Relieving Pose):

- Sit comfortably, hugging one knee to your chest at a time.

- Gently rock from side to side, massaging your lower back.

- Hold for 1-2 minutes while inhaling deeply.

- Reduces stress in the lower back and encourages relaxation.

119- Seated Forward Bend With Support:

- Sit with your legs outstretched, and use a pillow or cushion for support.

- Inhale to extend your spine, and exhale to fold forward.

- Hold for 2 minutes to allow your body to release stress.

- Stretches the spine and encourages relaxation.

120- Guided Relaxation Visualization:

- Close your eyes and imagine a serene place (such as a beach or forest).

- Spend 5 minutes immersing yourself in this fantastic world.

- Encourages mental relaxation and stress relief.

Tips:

Create a relaxing and tranquil environment.

Concentrate on every breath and sensation in your body.

Allow oneself to be free of any ideas or concerns.

Benefits:

Relaxes the neurological system and relieves tension.

Promotes mindfulness and bodily awareness.

Relaxes the muscles and produces a sense of calm.

Prepares the mind to slumber and rejuvenate.

DAY 21: Mindful Relaxation

Objective: Take part in a relaxing chair yoga session centered on awareness and relaxation.

Session highlights:

121- Deep Breathing Exercise:

- Sit comfortably and close your eyes.

- Inhale deeply through your nose for a count of 4.

- Exhale slowly through pursed lips for a count of six.

- Repeat for 3 minutes, focusing on your breathing.

122- Seated Body Scan Meditation:

- Bring attention to each area of your body, beginning with your toes.

- Notice any tightness or sensations and let them subside as you breathe.

- Move slowly up your body, until you reach the crown of your head.

- Takes about 5 minutes.

123- Chair Pawanmuktasana (Wind Relieving Pose):

- Sit comfortably, hugging one knee to your chest at a time.

- Gently rock from side to side, massaging your lower back.

- Hold for 1–2 minutes while breathing deeply.

- Reduces stress in the lower back and encourages relaxation.

124- Seated Forward Bend With Support:

- Sit with your legs outstretched, and use a pillow or cushion for support.

- Inhale to extend your spine, and exhale to fold forward.

- Hold for 2 minutes to allow your body to release stress.

- Stretches the spine and encourages relaxation.

125- Guided Relaxation Visualization:

- Close your eyes and imagine a serene place (such as a beach or forest).

- Spend 5 minutes immersing yourself in this fantastic world.

- Encourages mental relaxation and stress relief.

Tips:

Create a relaxing and tranquil environment.

Concentrate on every breath and sensation in your body.

Allow oneself to be free of any ideas or concerns.

Benefits:

Relaxes the neurological system and relieves tension.

Promotes mindfulness and bodily awareness.

Relaxes muscles and promotes a sense of tranquility.

Prepares the mind for rest and rejuvenation.

Week 4: Specialized Sequences and Conclusion

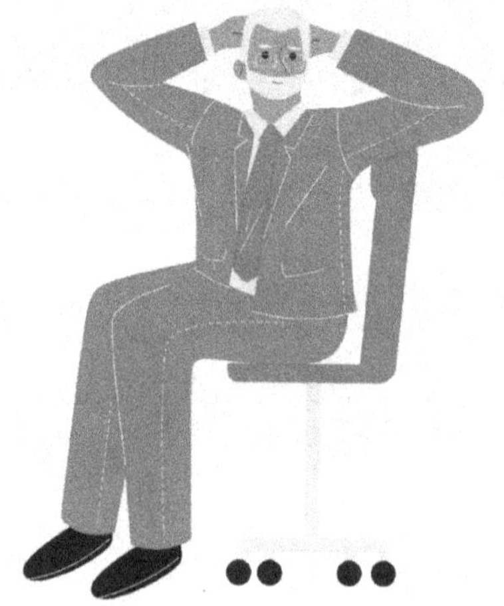

DAY 22: Full-Body Chair Flow: Strengthening Session

Objective: Perform a targeted chair yoga session to strengthen major muscle groups.

Session highlights:

126- Seated leg press:

- Sit with your feet flat on the floor and press one leg forward.

- Hold for 10 seconds then swap legs.

- Repeat for two minutes, alternating legs.

- Targets the quadriceps and increases leg strength.

127- Seated Push-ups:

- Sit at the edge of the chair, with your hands on the seat.

- Lift your body off the chair and then lower it back down.

- Perform 10-15 reps.

- Strengthens the chest, shoulders, and triceps.

128- Seated Knee Extensions:

- Sit tall, extend one leg straight, and hold for ten seconds.

- Lower one leg and switch to the other.

- Repeat for two minutes.

- Targets the quadriceps and improves knee stability.

129- Seated Twist With Resistance:

- Sit up straight and hold a resistance band.

- Twist your torso to one side and engage your core.

- Hold for 15 seconds per side.

- Strengthens core muscles and increases spinal mobility.

130- Chair triceps dips:

- Sit on the edge of the chair, with your hands on the sides.

- Slide off the chair, bend your elbows, and push back up.

- Perform 15-20 reps.

- Targets the triceps and increases arm strength.

Tips:

Maintain good form for all exercises.

Breathe consistently during the session.

Adjust the intensity to your fitness level.

Benefits:

Increases strength in the lower, core, and upper bodies.

Improves muscular tone and endurance.

Improves overall functional fitness.

Improves metabolism and fosters a sense of empowerment.

DAY 23: Seated Heart-Opening Poses: Comprehensive Renewal Routine

Objective: Enjoy a rejuvenating chair yoga exercise that incorporates flexibility, strength, and relaxation.

Session highlights:

131- Seated Neck and Shoulder Rolls:

- Sit comfortably and roll your shoulders in a circular motion.

- Gently move your neck side to side.

- Reduces tension in the neck and shoulders.

132- Chair Forward Fold and Breath Awareness:

- Sit with your feet flat, inhale deeply, and raise your arms overhead.

- Exhale and fold forward with a straight spine.

- Hold for 30 seconds, focusing on deep breathing.

- Stretches the entire back and promotes mindfulness breathing.

133- Dynamic Seated Warrior Flow.

- Sit on the edge of the chair and move between warrior-like gestures.

- Engage your core muscles and match your breathing and movement.

- Enhances strength, balance, and fluidity.

134- Seated Hip Openers and Twists:

- Sit tall and cross one ankle over the opposing knee.

- Gently twist toward the crossed knee.

- Hold for 20 seconds then switch sides.

- Releases hip tension and improves spinal flexibility.

135- Chair Sun Salutation Variation:

- Perform a modified sun salutation while seated.

- Flow between stretches and positions while connecting with your breath.

- Energizes the body and encourages general regeneration.

136- Sitting Mindful Breathing Meditation:

- Sit comfortably and close your eyes.

- Concentrate on your breath, inhaling and expelling deliberately.

- Practice for 5 minutes to develop a sensation of inner serenity.

- Promotes mental clarity and relaxation.

Tips:

Proceed slowly and thoughtfully through each pose.

Listen to your body and make adjustments as needed.

Accept the regenerating power of each movement.

Benefits:

The body and mind are renewed holistically.

Improved flexibility, strength, and balance.

Enhanced sense of inner calm and relaxation.

Prepares the body for restorative practices.

DAY 24: Seated Hip-Opening Flow - Targeted Muscle Activation

Objective: To improve strength and awareness, activate specific muscle areas with focused chair yoga techniques.

Session highlights:

137- Seated Glute Squeeze:

- Sit with a straight spine and squeeze your glutes together.

- Hold for 10 seconds Then release.

- Repeat for two minutes.

- Activates and strengthens gluteal muscles.

138- Chair Calf Raises:

- Sit with your feet flat on the floor.

- Lift heels off the ground and then lower them back down.

- Perform 15-20 reps.

- Strengthens the calf muscles and improves ankle stability.

139- Seated abdominal crunches:

- Sit tall and use your core muscles.

- Lean back slightly and bring your chest near your knees.

- Hold for 10 seconds and then return to an upright position.

- It strengthens the abdominal muscles.

140- Chair Bicep Curl:

- Hold a water bottle or a little weight in each hand.

- Sit up straight and curl the weights towards your shoulders.

- Perform 12 to 15 repetitions.

- Targets the biceps and increases arm strength.

140- Seated Shoulder Press:

- Hold weights in each hand at shoulder level.

- Press the weights overhead while extending your arms.

- Lower your back to shoulder height.

- Activates the shoulder muscles.

Tips:

To optimize effectiveness, perform each exercise with perfect technique.

To avoid strain, perform controlled motions.

During each activation, keep your focus on the targeted muscle group.

Benefits:

Improves muscular activation and strength in certain regions.

Improves muscular tone and definition.

Increases entire bodily awareness.

Promotes better posture and functional movement.

DAY 25: Seated Mountain Pose with Affirmations: Mindful Movement with Purpose

Objective: Practice mindful chair yoga practices to connect breath, movement, and intention.

Session highlights:

141- Seated Mountain Pose with Affirmation:

- Sit tall and keep your feet grounded.

- Inhale and raise your arms overhead.

- Exhale while repeating positive affirmations softly.

- Improves mindfulness and good intention.

142- Chair Twist for Gratitude:

- Sit with an erect spine and twist to one side.

- Inhale thankfulness; expel tension.

- Hold for 20 seconds then switch sides.

- Promotes thankfulness and relieves anxiety.

143- Seated Side Stretch for Presence:

- Inhale, raise one arm overhead, then lean to the side.

- Exhale, feeling the stretch along the torso.
- Exhale and feel the stretch throughout your torso.

- Hold for 15 seconds then switch sides.

- Improves bodily awareness and presence.

144- Dynamic Seated Warrior:

- Move through seated warrior-like exercises.

- Inhale during expansion, and exhale during contraction.

- Breathes and moves with purpose.

145- Mindful Seated Leg Extensions:

- Extend one leg at a time and feel the strain.

- Inhale as you expand, and exhale as you release.

- Perform for two minutes.

- Increases awareness of movement and breath synchrony.

Tips:

Concentrate on the current moment throughout each movement.

Breathe with deliberate intents.

Engage all of your senses in the encounter.

Benefits:

Purposeful movement helps to cultivate mindfulness.

Encourages a positive and intentional mindset.

Enhances the body-mind connection.

Promotes a sense of presence and thankfulness.

DAY 26: Seated Forward Bends and Inversions

Seated forward bends and inversions have a variety of benefits, including increased flexibility, reduced spinal tension, improved blood circulation, and a sensation of relaxation. These postures can also assist to reduce tension and anxiety while increasing focus and mental clarity.

Step 1: Prepare. Start in a comfortable seated position on your chair, feet flat on the ground. Sit upright, engage your core, and relax your shoulders. To find your core, take a few deep breaths.

Step 2: Seated Forward Bends.

146- Pose 1: Forward Fold.

Inhale and stretch your spine.

Exhale, hinge at your hips, and stretch forward to your toes.

Hold for 20-30 seconds while inhaling deeply.

Slowly return to the upright position.

147- Pose 2: Seated Wide-Legged Forward Bend.

Spread your legs wide, toes pointing forward.

Inhale and lift your chest.

Exhale and lean forward between your legs.

Hold for 20-30 seconds and feel the stretch in your inner thighs and lower back.

Inhale to get back up.

148 Step 3: Inversion in a Chair

Pose 3: Chair Forward Bend.

Sit on the edge of your chair, feet hip-width apart.

Inhale and stretch your spine.

Exhale and hinge at the hips, bringing your chest to your thighs.

Hold for 20-30 seconds while experiencing a slight stretch in your spine.

Inhale to get back to an upright position.

149 Pose 4: Modified Legs Up the Chair.

Sit comfortably and stretch your legs up the front of the chair.

Use your hands to support your lower back.

Hold for 20-30 seconds, enabling blood to return to your heart.

Gently lower your legs.

Step 4: Flow Sequence. Combine the seated forward bends and inversions to create a flowing sequence:

Sequence: Forward Fold (Pose 1), Chair Forward Bend (Pose 3), Seated Wide-Legged Forward Bend (Pose 2), and Modified Legs Up the Chair (Pose 4).

Step 5: Final Thoughts.

Take time to settle comfortably and breathe.

Recognize the benefits of the positions.

Express thanks for the time spent on self-care.

Practice these seated forward bends and inversions on a regular basis, paying attention to your body and adapting accordingly. As with any fitness routine, you should speak with a healthcare expert beforehand, especially if you have any pre-existing ailments. Enjoy the rejuvenating benefits of these chair yoga poses!

DAY 27: Seated Yin Yoga

Seated Yin Yoga emphasizes holding passive positions for long periods of time, which promotes deep stretching and relaxation. This technique focuses on connective tissues, increasing flexibility and promoting a contemplative state of mind.

150- Step 1: Set up Your Space

Find a quiet, comfortable spot to sit in your chair.

Make sure you will not be interrupted for the next 15-20 minutes.

Sit with your spine straight, shoulders relaxed, and your hands resting against your thighs.

151 Step 2: Start with centering breaths.

Close your eyes and take some calm, deep breaths.

Inhale through your nose, then exhale through your mouth, releasing tension with each breath.

Create a rhythmic breathing pattern to help soothe the nervous system.

Step three: Seated Forward Fold.

Inhale and stretch your spine.

Exhale, gradually hinge at your hips and fold forward.

Allow your hands to rest on the floor, or reach for your feet.

Hold the pose for 3–5 minutes, focusing on submitting to the stretch.

152- Step 4: Butterfly pose.

Bring the soles of your feet together and let your knees fall outward.

Sit up straight with your feet together.

Breathe deeply and relax into the stretch for 3-5 minutes.

153- Step 5: Supported Twist

Twist slightly to one side, using the chair's back as support.

Hold the twist for 2-3 minutes before switching to the other side.

Concentrate on gently releasing tightness in your spine.

154- Step 6: Seated Meditation.

Find a comfortable sitting position.

Close your eyes and focus your concentration inward.

Meditate for 5-7 minutes while watching your breath and allowing thoughts to pass without attachment.

155- Step 7: Closing

Gradually open your eyes.

Take time to savor the tranquility and calm.

Return to your day with a sense of peace and renewed vitality.

Seated Yin Yoga offers an opportunity for reflection and deep relaxation. Remember to listen to your body, and if a pose causes discomfort or agony, gradually ease out of it. Regular sitting Yin Yoga practice can help with flexibility, stress reduction, and overall well-being.

DAY 28: Celebration and Integration

Introduction: On this final day, we celebrate the end of the 28-day chair yoga journey and focus on incorporating the benefits into our daily lives. This session focuses on thankfulness, introspection, and looking forward to ongoing well-being.

156- Step 1: Gratitude Meditation

Start by sitting comfortably and shutting your eyes.

Consider how grateful you feel for taking the time to care for yourself.

Express gratitude for the body's resiliency and the path taken.

Reflect on the benefits of chair yoga in your life.

157- Step 2: Review Your Progress

Take time to reflect on the progress accomplished over the last 28 days.

Recognize increases in flexibility, strength, and overall well-being.

Celebrate any personal achievements made during the chair yoga program.

158- Step 3: Integrative Practices

Identify essential stances and sequences that resonate with you.

Consider incorporating these strategies into your daily routine or regular workout plan.

Consider how chair yoga can supplement other types of physical activity.

159- Step 4: Goal-Setting

Set realistic and attainable goals for your overall well-being.

Set future intentions, whether it's to attend regular chair yoga sessions or to experiment with other mindful activities.

160- Step 5: Mindful Breathing Exercise.

To center yourself, practice a short mindful breathing technique.

Inhale deeply and count to four. Exhale slowly to relieve tension.

Concentrate on the current moment and let go of any residual worry or anxiety.

161- Step 6: Ending Reflection

Close your eyes and take a few moments to think about your entire chair yoga experience.

Accept the sense of success and the pleasant effect on your body and mind.

Acknowledge your dedication to continual self-care and well-being.

162- Step 7: Celebration Ritual

Conclude the session by doing something special for yourself, such as eating a nutritious treat, going for a brief stroll, or participating in a favorite activity.

Celebrate the commitment to self-improvement and the path to a better living.

Congratulations on finishing the 28-day chair yoga program! May this celebration and integration period be the start of a long-term commitment to your well-being.

Contemplating the 28-Day Chair Yoga Expedition

As we reflect on our fulfilling 28-day adventure with Chair Yoga, we appreciate the transformations that have occurred. This one-of-a-kind adventure has been more than simply about postures; it has also been a deep investigation of well-being, resilience, and self-discovery.

During these 28 days, we've experimented with modified yoga postures, careful breathing, calming meditation, and the revitalizing effect of relaxation, all while sitting in a comfortable chair. It's not simply a physical trip; it's a comprehensive one that addresses our community's various needs.

As we reflect, we celebrate our accomplishments, including increased flexibility, a stronger core, and a better sense of balance. However, beyond the physical aspects, there is a deeper resonance—a journey of self-awareness, a connection with breath, and a pathway to inner tranquility.

Each day has served as a building brick, laying the groundwork for a sense of well-being that transcends beyond the mat. It is about incorporating the lessons learnt into daily life, cultivating mindfulness, and accepting the possibility of growth.

In this reflection, we recognize the collaborative energy of the chair yoga community. The combined dedication, encouragement, and mutual support have created a tapestry of unity and shared success. The 28-day voyage is more than simply a solo adventure; it is a collaborative quest for a more balanced and peaceful existence.

As we complete this thoughtful pause, let us carry forward the lessons learned, the resilience developed, and the sense of community that has grown. The 28-day chair yoga journey is not just a chapter, but a continuum—a pathway to prolonged well-being and a reminder that the voyage is ongoing, filled with possibilities for growth and self-discovery."

3 BONUS SEQUENCES

Sequence 1: Energizing Morning Flow.

Pose 1: Seated Cat-Cow Stretch.

Inhale, arch your back, and raise your chest.

Exhale, curve your spine, and bring your chin to your chest.

Step-by-Step Illustrated Guide:

Starting Position:

Sit comfortably on the edge of your chair, feet flat on the ground.

Place your hands on your knees or thigh.

Inhale: Arch your back.

Inhale deeply through your nose.

Lift your chest and let your spine to softly arch.

Keep your shoulders relaxed and drawn back.

Exhale: Round your spine.

Exhale through your mouth and engage your core.

Slowly circle your spine and bring your chin to your chest.

Feel the stretch across your upper back and between your shoulder blades.

Repeat the flow:

Continue the smooth transition between arcing and rounding.

Inhale the arch and open your chest.

For the round, exhale while engaging your core and bringing your chin to chest.

Coordinate with Breath:

Emphasize the coordination of breath and movement.

Inhale as you move to the arch.

Exhale as you assume the rounded position.

Repetition and awareness:

Repeat the sequence for 1-2 minutes at a slow speed.

Pay attention to your spine's movement and the sensation of the stretch.

Maintain a controlled and comfortable range of motion.

Tips:

Maintain a grounded and solid sitting position in the chair.

Adjust the degree of the stretch to your comfort level.

Relax your face muscles and keep a gentle gaze throughout the activity.

The Seated Cat-Cow Stretch mobilizes and warms up the spine, increasing flexibility and alleviating stress. This moderate sitting variant is ideal for those wishing to improve spinal mobility while seated.

Pose 2. Dynamic Arm Swings:

Swing your arms forth and back in a controlled motion.

Concentrate on activating the shoulders and warming up the upper body.

Step-by-Step Illustrated Guide:

Starting Position:

Sit comfortably in the chair, feet flat on the ground.

Maintain an erect stance with relaxed shoulders.

Relaxation and readiness:

Take a moment to relax your arms at your sides.

Prepare for the action by taking a soft, conscious breath.

Swing your arms forward.

Inhale deeply through your nose.

As you exhale, sweep both arms forward at the same time.

Keep the movement regulated.
Avoid any unexpected jerks.

Extend your arms comfortably in front of you, parallel to the floor.

Swing your arms backward.

Inhale again, then exhale while swinging both arms backward.

Imagine reaching behind you and opening your chest.

Maintain your shoulder blades engaged throughout this backward motion.

Repeat the dynamic swings:

Continue the rhythmic motion of swinging your arms forth and backward.

Maintain a consistent pace, synchronizing your movements with your breath.

To warm up the upper body, use a fluid, controlled pattern.

Focus on Shoulder Engagement:

Pay close attention to engaging your shoulders.

Feel the muscles contracting as you swing your arms forward and backward.

Avoid neck stress; maintain movements fluid and controlled.

Repetition and Duration:

Repeat the dynamic arm swings for 1-2 minutes, or until you feel comfortable.

Gradually extend the range of motion while maintaining control.

Tips:

Maintain a relaxed grip on the chair or allow your hands to hang gently during the swings.

Adjust the range of motion according to your comfort and flexibility.

Incorporate conscious and intentional breathing throughout the sequence.

Dynamic Arm Swings are an excellent warm-up for developing shoulder mobility and stimulating the upper body. This simple but powerful technique prepares your arms and shoulders for the following chair yoga poses.

Pose 3: Seated Sun Salutation.

Flow through modified sun salutations, including seated poses.

Emphasize breathing in unison with each movement.

Step-by-Step Illustrated Guide:

Starting Position:

Sit on the edge of your chair, keeping your spine erect.

Relax your shoulders and rest your hands on your knees or thighs.

Centering Breath:

Inhale deeply through your nose and raise your arms aloft.

Slowly exhale through your lips, bringing your hands to the heart center.

Mountain pose (tadasana):

Inhale, then extend your arms to the sides and overhead.

Reach upward to lengthen your spine.

Exhale and return your hands to the heart center.

Forward fold (uttanasana):

Inhale, then extend your arms forward and upward.

Exhale, hinge at the hips, and gradually fold forward.

Allow your hands to reach the floor or grab the chair legs.

Seated Forward Bend:

Inhale and elevate your torso to lengthen your spine.

Exhale, slowly round your back and reach for your feet.

Hold for a breath and feel the stretch in your lower back and hamstrings.

Repeat the mountain pose.

Inhale and return to an upright sitting position.

Extend your arms upward to stretch your spine.

Exhale and return your hands to the center of your heart.

Repeat the sequence:

Flow through the modified sun salutation 3-5 times.

Maintain a steady rhythm by coordinating each movement with your breathing.

Focus on Breath Synchronization:

Throughout the pattern, keep your breathing deep and intentional.

Inhale with upward movements, and exhale during forward folds and rounding.

Closing posture:

After the final round, sit down comfortably, close your eyes, and take a few deep breaths.

Recognize the invigorating benefits of the sitting sun salutation.

Tips:

Adjust the depth of the forward fold according to your flexibility.

Maintain seamless transitions between poses while remaining aware of your breath.

This seated sun salutation is a moderate warm-up that may be customized to your level of comfort.

Incorporate the Seated Sun Salutation into your chair yoga program to improve flexibility, increase circulation, and coordinate breath and movement.

Sequence 2: Stress Relief Midday Break

Pose 1: Chair Forward Bend.

Inhale and stretch the spine.

Exhale, hinge at the hips, and reach towards the floor.

Step-by-Step Illustrated Guide:

Starting Position:

Sit on the edge of your chair, feet flat on the ground.

Maintain a steady, grounded position.

Put your hands on your knees or thighs.

Centering Breath:

Inhale deeply through your nose, elevating your chest and stretching your spine.

Exhale softly through your lips, releasing tension and getting ready for the movement.

Inhale: Lengthen the spine.

Inhale and raise your arms overhead.

Extend your spine upward, stretching through the crown of your head.

Maintain a relaxed posture, with your shoulders away from your ears.

Exhale: Forward Bend.

Exhale, hinge at the hips, and lean forward with a flat back.

Allow your hands to reach the floor or grab the chair legs.

Maintain a mild stretch for your spine, hamstrings, and lower back.

Stretch & Hold:

Hold the forward bend for 20-30 seconds while breathing deeply.

Concentrate on elongating your spine and experiencing the stretch without effort.

Engage your core for stability.

Inhale - Return to the upright position:

Inhale again and slowly return to an upright seated position.

Lift your chest and lower your arms back to your sides.

Repeat the sequence:

Flow through the chair forward bend for 3-5 rounds, coordinating breath and movement.

Gradually raise the depth of the forward bend to your comfort level.

Closing posture:

After the last round, sit comfortably with a neutral spine.

Take a moment to enjoy the freedom and openness in your spine.

Tips:

Maintain a controlled and intentional movement throughout the sequence.

Adjust the depth of the forward bend to match your flexibility level.

Keep your neck in a neutral position to reduce tension.

The Chair Forward Bend helps to relax the spine, stretch the hamstrings, and increase flexibility. Add this posture to your chair yoga program for a gentle and effective way to enhance Spinal Mobility.

Pose 2: Gentle Neck and Shoulder Rolls.

Slowly roll your shoulders backward and forward.

Stretching your neck might help relieve tension.

Step-by-Step Illustrated Guide:

Starting Position:

Sit comfortably in the chair with a straight and relaxed spine.

posture your hands on your thighs or in a comfortable posture.

Centering Breath:

Inhale deeply through your nostrils and raise your shoulders to your ears.

Exhale slowly through your mouth to relieve tension in your neck and shoulders.

Shoulder Rolls Backward:

Inhale and roll both shoulders backward in a circular manner.

Roll your shoulders back and down after lifting them towards your ears.

Continue the circular motion to achieve a smooth and controlled movement.

Neck stretches:

Pause at the apex of the shoulder roll.

Inhale, then exhale, tilting your head gently to one side.

Feel a strain on the side of your neck.

Return your head to the center, then repeat on the opposite side.

Shoulder rolls forward:

Inhale deeply and roll your shoulders forward.

Lift your shoulders to your ears, then roll them forward and down.

Maintain a constant, controlled circular motion.

Neck stretches (continued):

Pause at the top of the forward shoulder roll.

Inhale and exhale as you bring your chin to your chest.

Feel a stretch on the back of your neck.

Lift your head back to the middle and repeat the stretch while looking up.

Repeat the sequence:

Continue with the gentle neck and shoulder rolls for 1-2 minutes.

Maintain a slow and deliberate tempo, concentrating on the release of tension.

Closing posture:

After finishing the rolls, sit with a neutral spine.

Take a moment to notice how your neck and shoulders feel more mobile and relaxed.

Tips:

Maintain smooth and steady movements, avoiding unexpected jerks.

Adjust the range of motion to your comfort level.

For maximum relaxation, incorporate deep breaths throughout the routine.

Gentle Neck and Shoulder Rolls are a simple yet effective approach to relieve stress, improve mobility, and increase upper-body comfort. Incorporate this relaxing pattern into your chair yoga regimen for moments of calm and peace.

Pose 3: Seated Twist.

Twist gently to either side, using the chair's back for support.

Concentrate on relieving tightness in the spine.

Step-by-Step Illustrated Guide:

Starting Position:

Sit comfortably and erect a spine on the chair.

Place your feet flat on the ground and your hands against your thighs.

Centering Breath:

Inhale deeply through your nose to stretch your spine.

Exhale slowly through your mouth to relieve tension and prepare for the twist.

Gently twist to the right.

Inhale deeply, sit tall, and stretch your spine.

Exhale and slowly shift your torso to the right.

Place your left hand on your right knee and your right hand on the chair's back for support.

Keep looking over your right shoulder.

Hold the twist:

Hold the twist for 20-30 seconds, keeping the spine extended.

Concentrate on gently releasing tightness from your spine.

Take deep breaths and feel the stretch in your mid back.

Return to center:

Inhale and slowly return to the center.

Sit tall and focus your spine.

Gently twist to the left:

Exhale and shift your torso to the left.

Place your right hand on your left knee and your left hand against the back of the chair.

Maintain a comfortable and controlled twist while gazing over your left shoulder.

Hold the twist (repeated):

Hold the twist for 20-30 seconds while breathing deeply.

Feel the gradual stretch down your spine, with an emphasis on tension release.

Breathe consciously, allowing the twist to feel comfortable.

Return to Center and Close Posture:

Inhale and return to the center, sitting tall.

Take a moment to sit with an elongated spine to reset your posture.

Tips:

Ensure that both feet are firmly planted on the ground during the twists.

To avoid tension on the lower back, use the chair's back as support.

Choose the depth of the twist based on your comfort level.

The Seated Twist is an excellent pose for relieving back stress, increasing mobility, and encouraging relaxation. Incorporate this easy twist into your chair yoga program to improve general spinal health.

Sequence 3: Evening Relaxation and Unwind

Pose 1: Seated Wide-Legged Forward Bend.

To stretch the spine, open your legs wide and inhale.

Exhale, hinge at the hips, and reach forward.

Step-by-Step Illustrated Guide:

Starting Position:

Sit comfortably in the chair, with your feet wider than hip width apart.

Maintain an erect posture by resting your hands on your thighs or knees.

Centering Breath:

Inhale deeply through your nose to stretch your spine.

Exhale slowly through your mouth to prepare for the forward bend.

Inhale: Lengthen the spine.

Inhale and spread your arms out to the sides.

Lift your chest, extending your spine upward.

Maintain a relaxed posture, with your shoulders away from your ears.

Exhale: Forward Bend.

Exhale, hinge at the hips, and lean forward with a flat back.

Allow your hands to reach the floor or grab the chair legs.

Maintain the length of your spine as you fold forward.

Stretch & Hold:

Hold the forward bend for 20-30 seconds while breathing deeply.

Feel the stretch on your inner thighs, hamstrings, and lower back.

Keep your gaze forward or slightly downward.

Inhale - Return to the upright position:

Inhale again and slowly return to an upright seated position.

Lift your chest and lower your arms back to your sides.

Repeat the sequence:

Flow through the seated wide-legged forward bend for 3-5 rounds.

To ensure a smooth and controlled exercise, coordinate each action with your breath.

Closing posture:

After the final round, maintain a neutral spine.

Take a moment to enjoy the freedom and openness in your hips and lower back.

Tips:

Maintain a controlled and intentional movement throughout the sequence.

Adapt the depth of the forward bend to your flexibility.

Keep your neck in a neutral position to reduce tension.

The Seated Wide-Legged Forward Bend is ideal for stretching the inner thighs and hamstrings while also increasing hip flexibility. Include this position in your chair yoga exercise to improve lower body mobility and provide a gentle relaxation for the spine.

Pose 2 (Supported Legs Up the Chair):

Sit at the edge of the chair, extend your legs up, and support your lower back.

Promote blood circulation and moderate inversion.

Step-by-Step Illustrated Guide:

Starting Position:

Sit on the edge of your chair, back straight, shoulders relaxed.

Extend your legs straight in front of you, heels resting on the ground.

Centering Breath:

Inhale deeply through your nose to stretch your spine.

Slowly exhale through your lips, preparing for the supported legs up the chair.

Sit at the edge.

Scoot to the front of the chair, keeping your lower back toward the edge.

Inhale - Lift the legs:

Inhale and pull both legs up, stretching them toward the ceiling.

Keep your knees slightly bent if necessary to maintain comfort.

Engage your core to support the lift.

Support the lower back.

Put your hands on your lower back for further support.

Adjust your position to maintain comfort and stability.

This supportive position eases tension on the lower back.

Hold the position:

Hold the legs up for 20-30 seconds, or until you feel comfortable.

Focus on deep breathing to promote relaxation and gentle inversion.

Experience the stretch in your hamstrings and the renewing effect on your legs.

Gradual descent:

Exhale and slowly lower your legs back to the floor.

Maintain control throughout the drop by utilizing your core muscles.

Repeat the sequence:

Perform the supported leg up the chair for 3-5 rounds.

Adjust the intensity to your flexibility and comfort level.

Closing posture:

After the final round, sit back and relax with an upright spine.

Take time to see the improved blood circulation and rejuvenation.

Tips:

To maintain stability, move slowly and with control.

Listen to your body and avoid overextending your legs if it hurts.

Use the chair's edge as support to ensure a safe and comfortable practice.

Supported Legs Up the Chair is an excellent pose for improving blood circulation, gently inverting the body, and stretching the legs.

Incorporate this position into your chair yoga program for a refreshing and revitalizing experience.

Pose 3: Guided Relaxation Meditation.

Close your eyes and take deep, relaxing breaths.

Guide your mind on a relaxing journey, reducing stress from head to toe.

Step-by-Step Illustrated Guide:

Find a comfortable sitting position:

Sit comfortably in the chair, back straight and shoulders relaxed.

posture your hands on your thighs or in a comfortable posture.

Centering Breath:

Inhale deeply through your nose to fill your lungs with air.

Exhale slowly through your mouth to relieve any tension or stress.

Close your eyes.

Gently close your eyes to achieve inner focus.

Allow your gaze to soften and focus your attention inside.

Deep, calm breaths:

Inhale deeply and count to four.

Exhale softly, releasing any tension or discomfort.

Repeat the rhythmic breathing to induce a state of calm.

Mindful Body Scan:

Focus your concentration on your head. Inhale deeply, envisioning calmness spreading across your scalp and forehead.

Exhale, releasing tension and allowing your jaw to soften.

Move down to your neck and shoulders. Inhale and feel the breath relax any tension.

Exhale, releasing any tension or stiffness in your neck and shoulders.

Continue your focused body scan, taking in your arms, chest, back, belly, and hips. Inhale relaxation, expel stress.

Concentrate on your legs, from the thighs to the calves and finally to your feet. Inhale serenity and exhale any remaining stress.

Imagery and visualization:

Imagine a peaceful area, such as a beach or a forest.

Inhale the peace of that area and exhale any leftover concerns.

Affirmations and positivity:

Incorporate positive affirmations like "I am calm," or "I am at peace."

Repeat these affirmations with each breath to maintain a positive outlook.

Gradual Awareness:

Gradually become conscious of your surroundings.

Gently open your eyes, bringing a sense of calm into the present.

Final Moments:

Take a few seconds to enjoy the feelings of serenity and relaxation.

Recognize the silence within and embrace its rejuvenating influence.

Tips:

Adjust the pace of your breath and the duration of the meditation to your liking.

Use calming imagery that speaks to you for a more personalized experience.

Practice this guided relaxation meditation on a regular basis to improve stress reduction and mental health.

Guided Relaxation Meditation is an effective strategy for reducing stress, increasing mindfulness, and creating a deep sense of relaxation. Incorporate this meditation into your chair yoga practice for moments of relaxation and refreshment.

Use these supplementary routines according to your schedule and energy levels. Whether you need an energetic start, stress relief during the day, or a soothing evening routine, these sequences are designed to improve your chair yoga experience and general well-being.

Appendix

&

References

Resources for Continued Exploration

"Chair Yoga Basics" by Lili Audrey

A comprehensive guide to the fundamentals of chair yoga, offering in-depth insights into postures, modifications, and the transformative potential of this practice.

"Mindful Breathing: A Journey Within" by Laura Danfur

Delve into the art of mindful breathing with this insightful resource, exploring techniques to enhance relaxation, focus, and overall well-being.

"The Healing Power of Meditation" by Justin Nicholas

Discover the profound benefits of meditation on physical and mental health, providing practical guidance for integrating meditation into daily life.

"Chair Yoga for Every Body" DVD Series

A visual companion to your chair yoga journey, offering guided sessions led by experienced instructors, catering to various levels and abilities.

"The Science of Yoga" by William J. Broad

Explore the scientific aspects of yoga, gaining a deeper understanding of its impact on the body and mind, and how it can contribute to overall health.

Dear Value Reader

As we near the end of our trip together, I'd like to convey my heartfelt gratitude for choosing this chair yoga instruction. If even one reader finds value, comfort, or inspiration in these pages, I consider it a great success.

Your good feedback has the ability to uplift and encourage. Your remarks become a beacon, directing others to discover the benefits of chair yoga. Your feedback not only drives my motivation, but also demonstrates the positive influence this practice may have on our well-being.

Remember, your words are more than just a review; they are confirmation that the work put into this book has made a significant difference. Your encouragement inspires me to keep generating content that resonates and encourages your journey to wellness.

Thank you for being a part of this community. May your words inspire others to embark on their chair yoga journey, discovering the joy and well-being it brings.

Wishing you continued health, happiness, and a harmonious journey ahead.

With gratitude,
Prancis Nova

www.ingramcontent.com/pod-product-compliance
Lightning Source LLC
Chambersburg PA
CBHW050811260726
48660CB00004B/1370